Visual fields via the visual pathway

Visual fields via the visual pathway

Fiona Rowe

PhD, DBO, CGLI CertEd

Lecturer in Orthoptics, Division of Orthoptics, University of Liverpool
Honorary Research Associate, Department of Orthoptics and
Ophthalmology, Warrington Hospital

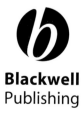

Blackwell
Publishing

Blackwell Publishing Ltd
Editorial offices:
Blackwell Publishing Ltd, 9600 Garsington Road, Oxford OX4 2DQ, UK
    Tel: +44 (0)1865 776868
Blackwell Publishing Inc., 350 Main Street, Malden, MA 02148-5020, USA
    Tel: +1 781 388 8250
Blackwell Publishing Asia Pty Ltd, 550 Swanston Street, Carlton, Victoria 3053, Australia
    Tel: +61 (0)3 8359 1011

The right of the Author to be identified as the Author of this Work has been asserted in accordance with the Copyright, Designs and Patents Act 1988.

First published 2006 by Blackwell Publishing Ltd

ISBN-13: 978-14051-1525-4
ISBN-10: 1-4051-1525-4

Library of Congress Cataloging-in-Publication Data

Rowe, Fiona J.
    Visual fields via the visual pathway/Fiona Rowe.
        p. cm.
    Includes bibliographical references.
    ISBN-13: 978-14051-1525-4 (pbk. : alk. paper)
    ISBN-10: 1-4051-1525-4 (pbk. : alk. paper)
    1. Perimetry. 2. Visual Fields. 3. Visual Pathways. I. Title.
    [DNLM: 1. Perimetry. 2. Visual Fields. 3. Visual Pathways.
WW 145 R878v 2006]
RE79.P4R69 2006
617.7′5- -dc22

A catalogue record for this title is available from the British Library

Set in 10/12 pt Sabon
by Newgen Imaging Systems (P) Ltd, Chennai, India
Printed and bound in India
by Replika Press Pvt, Ltd, Kundli

The publisher's policy is to use permanent paper from mills that operate a sustainable forestry policy, and which has been manufactured from pulp processed using acid-free and elementary chlorine-free practices. Furthermore, the publisher ensures that the text paper and cover board used have met acceptable environmental accreditation standards.

For further information on Blackwell Publishing, visit our website:
www.blackwellpublishing.com

Contents

Colour plates appear after p. 78

List of Tables

List of Figures

Unless otherwise stated the right visual field is displayed above the left visual field result, or to the right side of the left visual field result. **Note:** the blind spot appears on the right side of central fixation within the right visual field, and on the left side of central fixation within the left visual field.

List of Colour Plates

Colour plates appear after p. 78.

Preface

Visual Fields via the Visual Pathway presents the varying visual field deficits occurring with lesions of the visual pathway. The main content is structured such that the visual pathway is traced anatomically from front to back, and each section of the visual pathway has its own dedicated chapter.

The chapters are clearly structured and comprise an outline of anatomy, pathology and signs and symptoms, plus visual field defects specifically associated with that part of the visual pathway. Each chapter is supplemented by numerous illustrations of visual field results, neuroimaging scans and/or line drawings; colour plates of associated fundus images are also provided.

In addition, chapters are provided on the basic theory of visual field assessment, methodology, aids to differential diagnosis, artefacts of visual field results and a glossary of terms used in visual field assessment. References and further reading lists are provided for each chapter, containing key articles and up-to-date literature.

This textbook has been written to provide a guide for the multi-disciplinary eye care team: ophthalmologists, orthoptists, optometrists, ophthalmic technicians and ophthalmic nurse practitioners. Its clinical content for both text and illustrations is particularly relevant for the practitioner.

Unless otherwise stated the right visual field is displayed above the left visual field result, or to the right side of the left visual field result. **Note:** the blind spot appears on the right side of central fixation within the right visual field, and on the left side of central fixation within the left visual field.

Disclosure

Dr Rowe has no financial or commercial interest in either Goldmann perimeters or Humphrey visual field analysers.

Acknowledgements

Thanks are due to my colleagues at the University of Liverpool (Division of Orthoptics) for their support, and to colleagues at Warrington Hospital (Department of Ophthalmology) for their support when compiling many of the illustrations. Special thanks are due to colleagues at Addenbrooke's Hospital, Cambridge, and in particular to Tracy Crowley, for help in improving the quality of a number of visual field results. I am very grateful to Carl Zeiss Ltd (Humphrey Instruments) and in particular to Dr Patella, for permission to reproduce illustrations* and for general advice in relation to the Humphrey visual field analyser. Lastly, many thanks to Caroline Connelly and her team at Blackwell Publishing for their input to this text.

*Heijl A, Patella VM (2002) *The field analyzer primer. Essential perimetry.* 3rd edition. Dublin, CA, Carl Zeiss Meditec; Haley MJ (1987) *The field analyzer primer.* 2nd edition. San Leandro, CA, Humphrey systems

Dedication

This book is dedicated to my family.

'The family is one of nature's masterpieces.'

George Santayana

Chapter 1

Field of vision and visual pathway

Visual field assessment is the process by which the boundaries of the visual field are plotted and the field within the peripheral boundaries is determined to be intact. Assessment of the visual field has been undertaken in varying ways since the blind spot was first documented by Mariotte in the seventeenth century. The outer boundaries of the visual field were assessed by Young and Purkinje in the nineteenth century. However, the first clinical measurement of the visual field was not made until the 1850s and this was achieved by von Graefe.

Varying methodologies have been developed for the assessment of the field of vision since the nineteenth century. In 1889, Bjerrum introduced a tangent screen for assessment of the visual field which currently retains his name. This predominantly assessed the central visual field. The Arc perimeter was introduced by Aimark in the 1930s which had the advantage of being able to plot the peripheral visual field. This was followed by the introduction of the Goldmann perimeter in 1945 which today remains in widespread use and continues to be of considerable clinical value.

The Friedmann perimeter was the first quantitative static measurement introduced in 1966 and assessed the central visual field. Automated perimetry was introduced in the 1970s with the subsequent development of a myriad of different automated perimeters with many testing programmes which today provide accurate and reliable visual fields with the advantage of statistical analysis of results and computer storage of patient files. The automated perimeter most commonly in current use in hospital practice is the Humphrey field analyser (Humphrey Systems, Dublin, CA).

General anatomy of the visual system

The hill of vision is a map of the visual sensitivity across the visual field, usually in three dimensions. A one dimension representation usually takes a horizontal section bisecting the optic disc and fovea (Fig. 1.1). The central peak of the hill equates to the fovea and is typically the area of highest sensitivity. Sensitivity decreases towards the periphery of the visual field. The normal monocular visual field extends 50–60 degrees superiorly, 60 degrees nasally, 70–75 degrees inferiorly and 90–100 degrees temporally (Kanski & McAllister 1989; Stamper *et al.* 1999). The extent

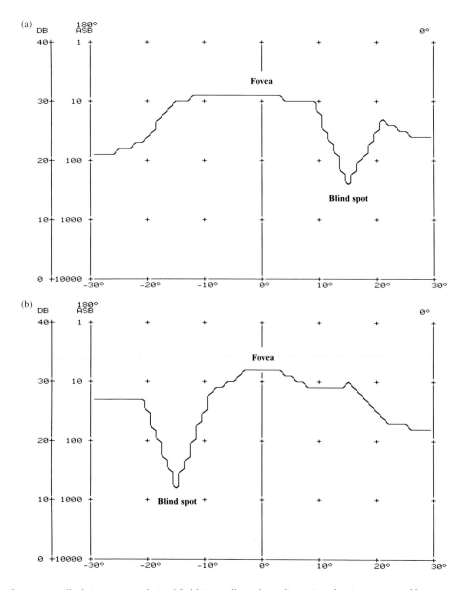

Figure 1.1 Hill of vision. Map of visual field is usually in three dimensions but is represented here in one dimension. The central peak has the highest sensitivity and represents the fovea. Sensitivity decreases towards the periphery of the visual field.

of visual field will vary with stimulus size, and the extent measured with a Goldmann I4e or $\frac{3}{4}$ mm white target is regarded as normal (Fig. 1.2). As the optic disc has no retinal photoreceptors, it forms the blind spot of the visual field.

The visual field is produced by retinal stimulation of each eye and relates to what is seen by the individual whilst maintaining steady fixation, i.e. it is the perceived vision of an individual. Retinal images are projected to a position opposite the area of retina stimulated; for example, objects that stimulate nasal retina are situated in

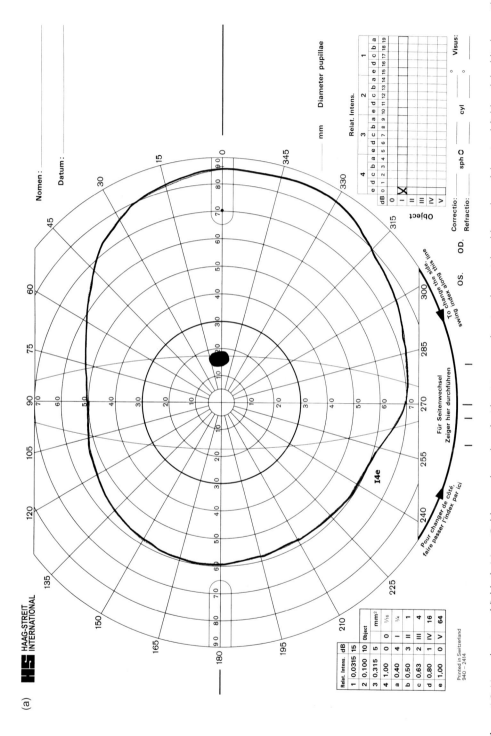

Figure 1.2 Normal extent of field of vision. Goldmann chart plotted with a I4e target showing the peripheral boundary of the visual field and the blind spot. The extent of peripheral boundary is age dependent: (a) 20 year old; (b) 60 year old.

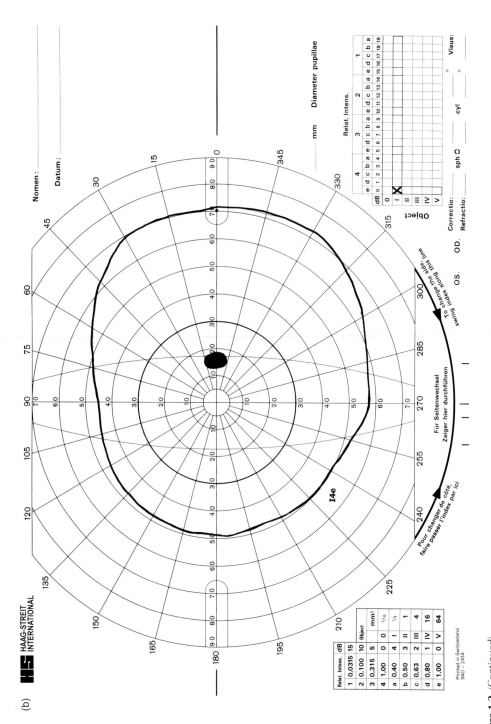

Figure 1.2 (Continued)

the temporal visual field and objects that stimulate inferior retina are situated in the superior visual field.

A high percentage of nerve fibres arise from the macular area of the retina and pass directly to the optic disc (papillomacular bundle). Nerve fibres located further temporally in the peripheral retina (nasal field of vision) must arc above and below the macular fibres to enter the optic disc superiorly and inferiorly. Nerve fibres on the nasal side of the optic disc (temporal field of vision) pass directly to the nasal border.

Once in the optic nerve, the macular fibres move to a central position with superior retinal fibres above and inferior retinal fibres below. Temporal and nasal nerve fibres retain their temporal and nasal location within the optic nerve.

On reaching the optic chiasm, the temporal nerve fibres maintain their temporal position whilst nasal nerve fibres (both central and peripheral) decussate. Ipsilateral temporal nerve fibres and contralateral nasal nerve fibres regroup in the optic tracts, but again with superior fibres retaining a more superior location to the inferior fibres.

Nerve fibres are distributed in a complicated multi-layered arrangement in the lateral geniculate nucleus of the lateral geniculate body, with macular fibres distributed throughout the nucleus. Ipsilateral and contralateral peripheral nerve fibres are located in different layers of the nucleus. There is a synapse of nerve fibres in the lateral geniculate body.

Fibres leaving the lateral geniculate body fan out to form the optic radiations, many of which pass directly posterior to the visual cortex. A proportion, however, initially pass anteriorly and laterally before turning posterior towards the visual cortex.

Within the striate visual cortex (V1) the macular fibres terminate on the tip of the occipital lobe (occipital pole), whilst the more peripheral fibres terminate more anteriorly. The most peripheral fibres relating to the monocular crescent of each eye are the most anteriorly represented. Superior fibres are on the upper lip of the calcarine fissure, whilst inferior fibres are on the lower lip. Figure 1.3 represents the afferent visual pathway.

Visual field defect types

Altitudinal visual field defect (Fig. 1.4)

This involves two quadrants of either the superior or inferior visual field and is typically seen in ischaemic optic neuropathies. The defect precisely respects the horizontal meridian. The sharp horizontal separation occurs because there is a clear demarcation between superior and inferior nerve fibres temporal to the macula and nasal to the optic disc.

Severe hypotension, sudden haemorrhage and rapid development of anaemia may be responsible for simultaneous bilateral ischaemic optic neuropathies with altitudinal visual field defects. They may also be due to bilateral symmetric involvement at a cortical level, including bilateral lesions affecting the occipital lobe (Heller-Bettinger *et al.* 1976; Miller & Newman 1999).

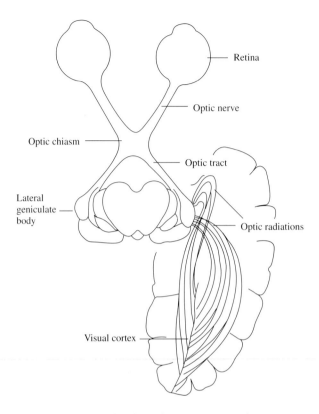

Figure 1.3 Afferent visual pathway. Visual pathway from retina to visual cortex.

Arcuate visual field defect (Fig. 1.5)

This is caused by selective damage to the superior or inferior retinal nerve fibre bundles as they enter the optic nerve head and is typical of glaucoma. However, such visual field defects are also seen in optic neuritis, ischaemic optic neuropathy and congenital optic disc drusen.

Temporally, the defect is narrow because all of the nerve fibre bundles converge on the optic disc. The defect spreads out on the nasal side, but typically arcs over central fixation. All complete arcuate scotomas extend to the horizontal meridian producing a nasal step, assuming there is differing involvement of the superior and inferior visual fields.

Hemianopia (Fig. 1.6)

A hemianopia is a complete defect involving one half of the visual field. A heterony-mous hemianopia involves opposite sides of the visual field (e.g. lesions of the optic chiasm typically produce bitemporal heteronymous hemianopias). A homonymous hemianopia involves the same side of the visual field in each eye (e.g. lesions of the retrochiasmal pathways typically produce homonymous hemianopias).

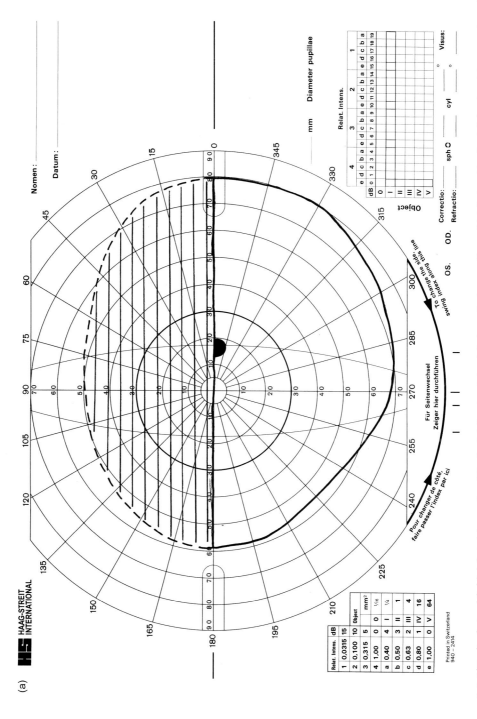

Figure 1.4 Altitudinal visual field defect: (a) superior altitudinal defect involving inferior retinal nerve fibres; (b) inferior altitudinal defect involving superior retinal nerve fibres.

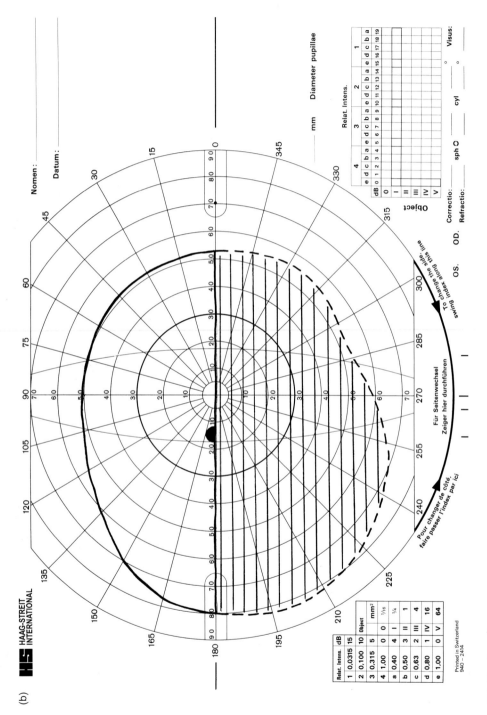

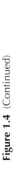

Figure 1.4 (Continued)

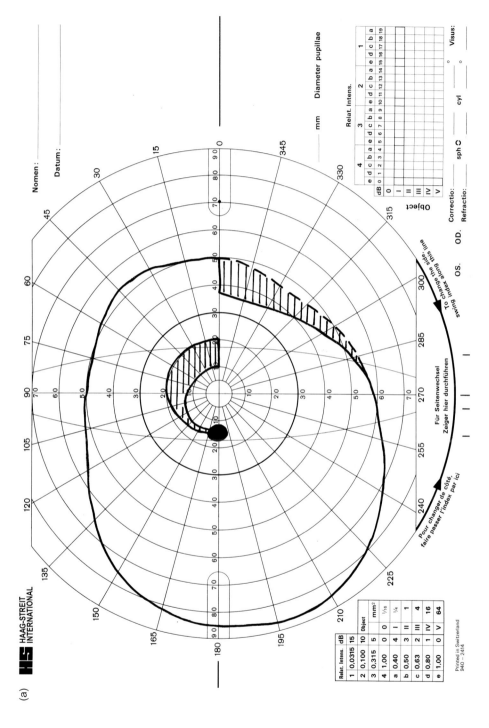

Figure 1.5 Arcuate visual field defect: (a) superior arcuate defect with inferior nasal step; (b) inferior arcuate defect.

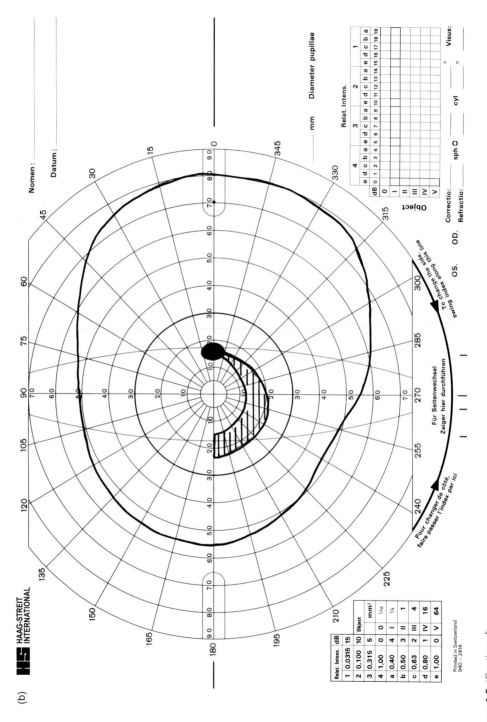

Figure 1.5 (Continued)

Quadrantanopia (Fig. 1.7)

This is a complete defect involving a quadrant of each visual field. Heteronymous quadrantanopia involves opposite sides of the visual field and either superior or inferior quadrants. Homonymous quadrantanopias involve the same side of the visual field in each eye and either superior or inferior quadrants. These may be produced by temporal, parietal or occipital lobe lesions.

Scotoma

A scotoma is an absolute or relative area of depressed visual sensitivity surrounded by normal vision. In an absolute scotoma all vision is lost, whereas in a relative scotoma a variable amount of vision remains. Scotomas may be central, paracentral or caecocentral in type.

A central scotoma only involves fixation (Fig. 1.8a). The scotoma can be relative or absolute depending on the severity of the lesion. A central scotoma typically occurs in optic neuritis, although it can also be caused by ischaemic and compressive optic nerve lesions.

A paracentral scotoma (Fig. 1.8b) involves an area of visual field away from fixation and tends to be elongated circumferentially along the course of the optic nerve fibres within the central 30 degrees. It may be seen in glaucoma or lesions affecting the optic disc such as papilloedema.

A caecocentral scotoma (Fig. 1.8c) extends from fixation to the blind spot and is caused by disease of the papillomacular bundle. It typically occurs in toxic optic neuropathies and Leber's optic neuropathy. Congenital optic disc pits associated with serous detachment of the macula may also produce a similar defect. Bilateral caecocentral scotomas may be due to toxic amblyopia, optic neuritis, Leber's optic neuropathy or intrinsic optic nerve tumours.

Sector-shaped (wedge) visual field defect (Fig. 1.9)

These visual field defects start as small scotomas on the temporal side of the visual field and end as complete sectorial loss.

Parameters and variables in visual field assessment

There are a number of parameters that must be considered when undertaking quantitative visual field assessment:

(1) The size of stimulus
(2) Luminance intensity
(3) Anatomical features
(4) Interference with perception of stimuli
(5) Patient ability
(6) Examination technique.

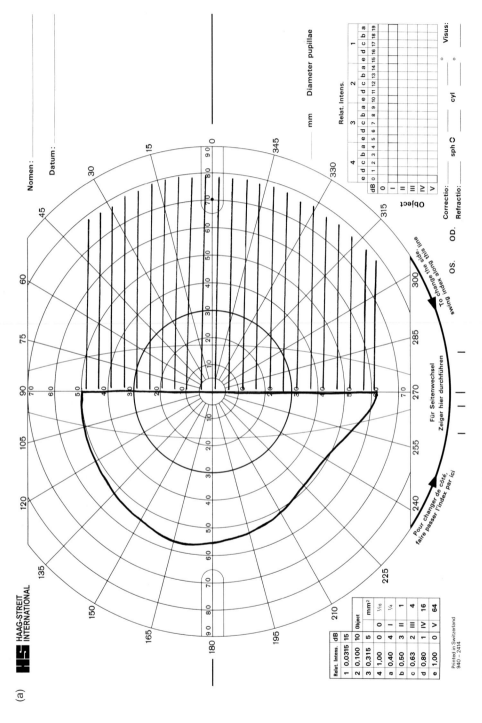

(a)

Figure 1.6 Hemianopia: (a) bitemporal hemianopia; (b) homonymous hemianopia.

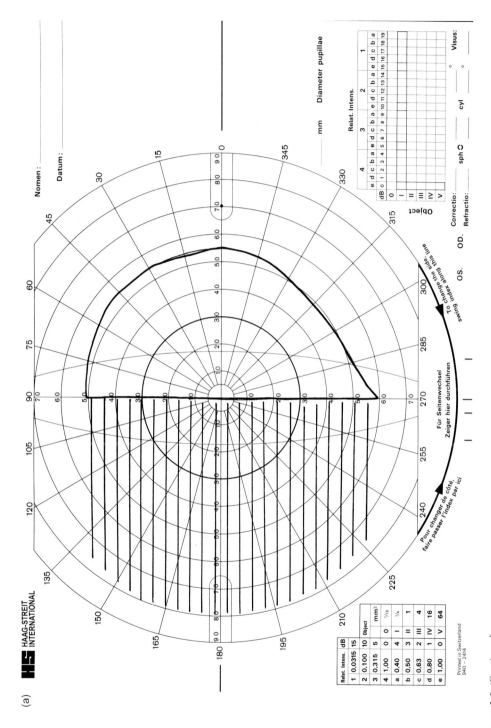

Figure 1.6 (Continued)

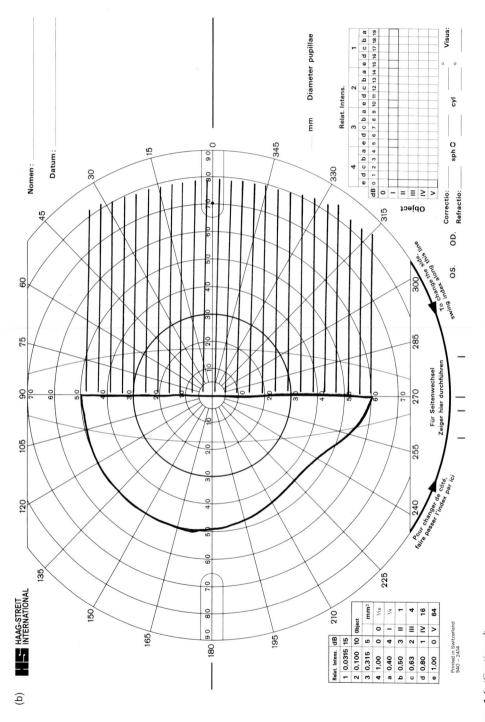

Figure 1.6 (Continued)

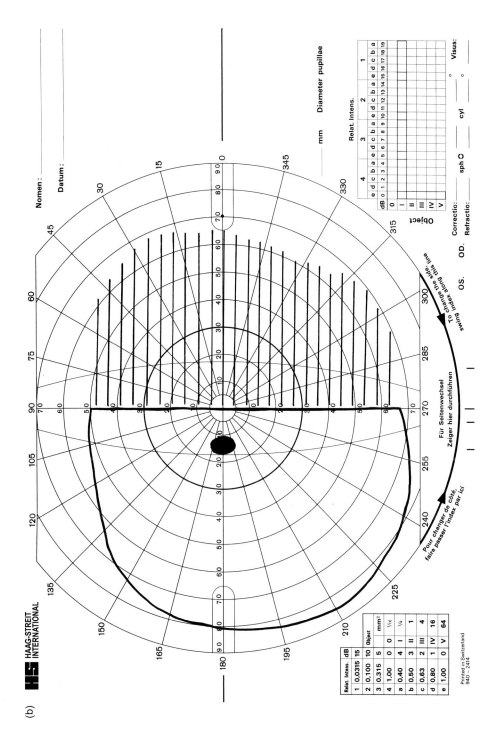

Figure 1.6 (Continued)

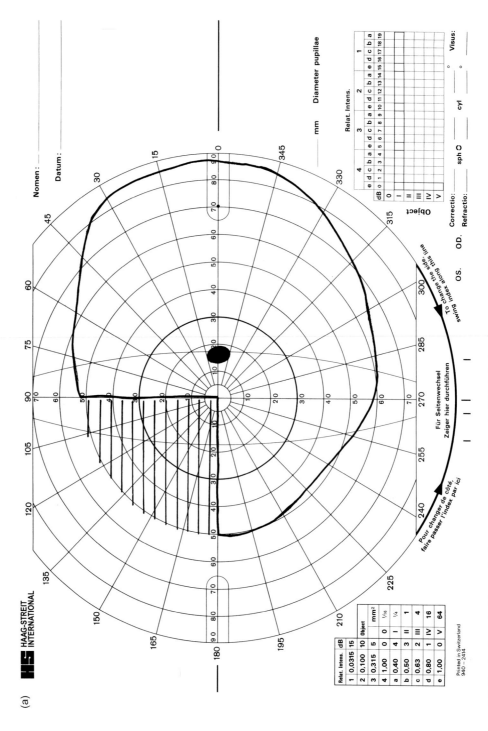

Figure 1.7 Quadrantanopia: (a) superior homonymous quadrantanopia; (b) inferior homonymous quadrantanopia.

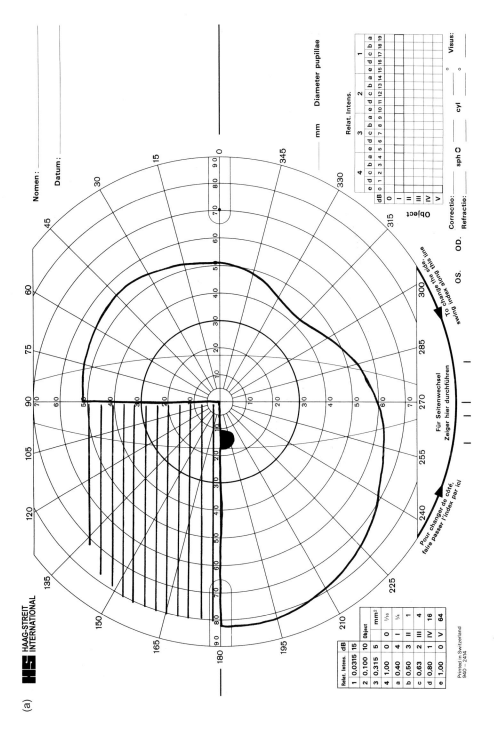

Figure 1.7 (Continued)

(b)

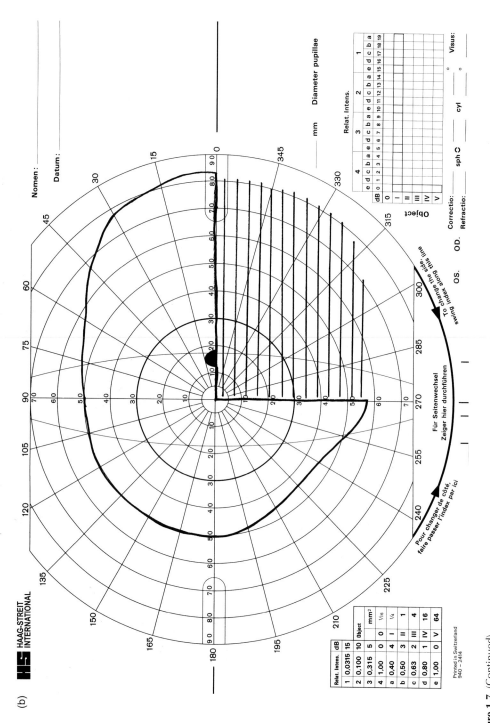

Figure 1.7 (Continued)

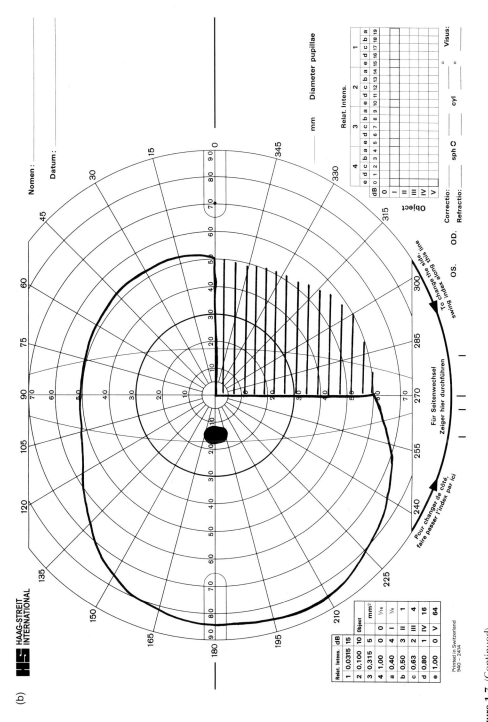

Figure 1.7 (Continued)

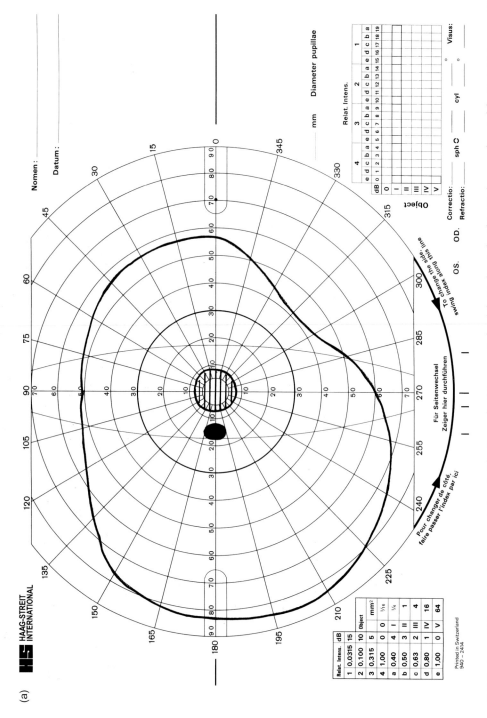

Figure 1.8 Scotomas: (a) central – involvement of central fixation only; (b) paracentral – defect is located within 30 degrees of central fixation; (c) caecocentral – central fixation is involved with extension of the defect to the blind spot.

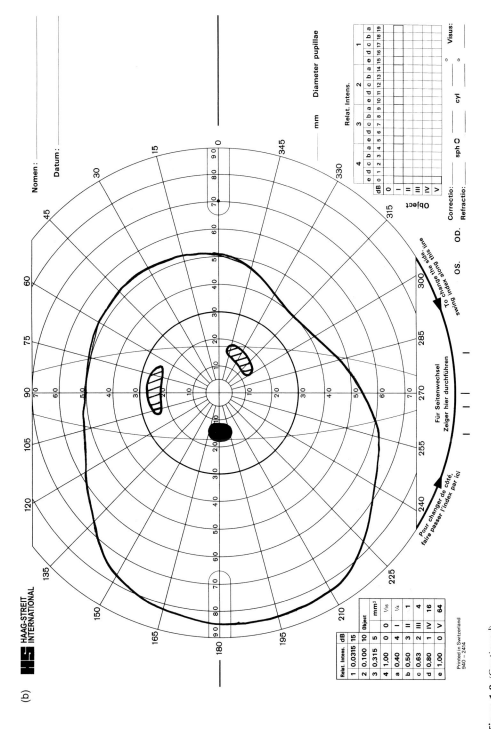

Figure 1.8 (Continued)

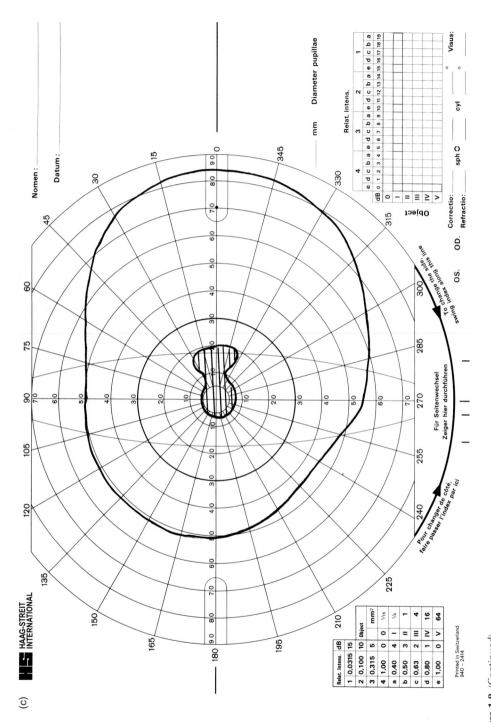

Figure 1.8 (Continued)

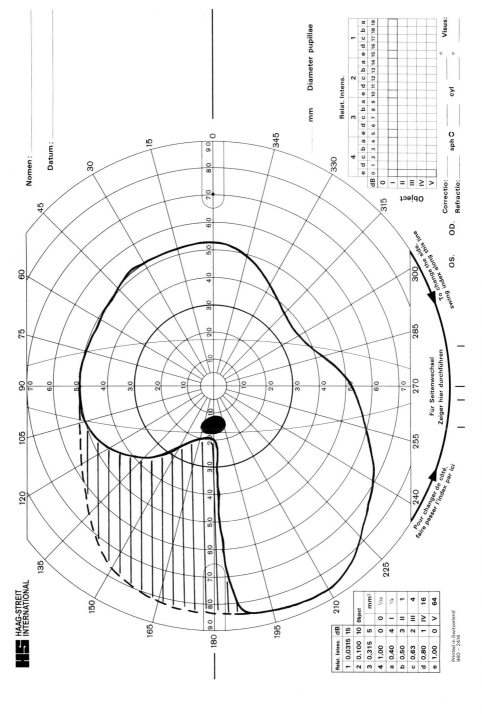

Figure 1.9 Sector-shaped (wedge) visual field defect. Temporal defect extends to the blind spot.

Table 1.1 Size and intensity of targets in Goldmann perimetry.

Stimulus[a]	Intensity		Size of target (mm^2)
	Apostilb	Decibel	
V4e	1000	0	64
IV4e	315	5	16
III4e	100	10	4
II4e	31.5	15	1
I4e	10	20	1/4
I3e	3.15	25	1/4
I2e	1	30	1/4
I1e	0.315	35	1/4

[a] These eight standard stimuli are used to allow continuity of testing and interpretation.

The size of stimulus can be varied in that stimuli can be presented in sizes I to V in both Humphrey automated and Goldmann manual perimetry ($\frac{1}{4}$ mm^2 to 64 mm^2; Table 1.1). Size III stimulus is standardly set for automated perimetry (4 mm^2). The size of stimuli remains constant in Humphrey automated perimetry, thereby providing consistent stimuli. Stimulus size is varied during testing in manual Goldmann perimetry when plotting peripheral and central isopters.

The sensitivity of the visual field is expressed in luminance or light intensity units. Luminance units are candelas per square metre (cd/m^2). Light intensity is expressed as an apostilb which is an absolute unit of light measurement equal to 0.1 millilamberts (1 cd/m^2 equals 3.14 asb). The range of retinal light sensitivity measured by visual field assessment is expressed in log units with a base of 10. In perimetry, stimulus intensity for visual field assessment is represented in decibel values which equal $\frac{1}{10}$ th of a log unit (10 decibels equals 1 log unit) and allows larger numbers to be expressed as smaller numerical units. Therefore changes in sensitivity are more easily detected (0 decibels = 1000 apostilb = 300 cd/m^2).

The luminous intensity of the stimulus in automated visual field assessment may be altered from 0 to 51 decibels, providing a wide range of brightness levels for stimuli to completely assess the threshold of all visual field areas. The relative luminance between background and stimulus will alter sensitivity. In Goldmann and Humphrey perimetry the background illumination is set at 31.5 apostilb. This standard calibration is necessary for test/retest repeatability. The area of retina stimulated will provide different responses to stimuli, i.e. peripheral retinal responses have lower luminance sensitivity than central retinal responses.

There are a number of external variables that must be considered with regard to the visual field result. These include anatomical features of the face (e.g. prominent brow or nose), interference with ocular media and perception of stimuli (e.g. ptosis, miotic pupil, uncorrected refractive error, cataract), attention and age of the patient, and technique of the examiner (explanation of the test and patient set-up) (Haas *et al.* 1986; Johnson *et al.* 1989).

Protruding facial features such as lids and brows may provide spurious visual field defects, often in the superior visual field. Where there is ptosis, the lid should be taped to prevent it blocking stimuli presentation.

Miosis depresses the visual field and can exaggerate the size and depth of existing visual field defects. Pupil diameter less than 2 mm produces visual field loss as pupil constriction dims both the intensity of the stimulus and the intensity of the background. This is a problem when assessing patients on miotics for glaucoma (Mikelberg *et al.* 1987; Lindenmuth *et al.* 1989).

Refractive errors, if uncorrected, can result in refractive scotomas with enlarged blind spots and enlargement of other visual field defects. There is also a depression of sensitivity in the visual field. Defocus effectively enlarges the stimulus size but will reduce the luminance (Atchison 1987; Henson & Morris 1993). Refractive errors greater than 1 dioptre should be corrected and the prescription given according to the patient's age and instrument optics. Incorrect spectacle corrections can also cause artefacts due to reduced light sensitivity which may produce local or generalised visual field loss.

Abnormalities that interfere with media clarity reduce illumination; therefore sensitivity within the visual field will be generally depressed and existing visual field defects exaggerated (Guthauser *et al.* 1987).

Age gradually depresses the visual field sensitivity. Light-difference sensitivity decreases with age partly due to age-related loss of nerve fibres (Balazsi *et al.* 1984) and increased condensation of the media.

References

Atchison DA (1987) Effect of defocus on visual field measurement. *Ophthalmic and Physiological Optics*, 7: 259

Balazsi AG, Rootman J, Drance SM, Schulzer M, Douglas GR (1984) The effect of age on the nerve fibre population of the human optic nerve. *American Journal of Ophthalmology*, **97**: 760

Guthauser U, Flammer J, Niesel P (1987) Relationship between cataract density and visual field damage. *Documenta Ophthalmologica Proceedings Series*, **49**: 39

Haas A, Flammer J, Schneider U (1986) Influence of age on the visual fields of normal subjects. *American Journal of Ophthalmology*, **101**: 199

Heller-Bettinger I, Kepes JJ, Preskorn SH, Wurster JB (1976) Bilateral altitudinal anopia caused by infarction of the calcarine cortex. *Neurology*, **26**: 1176

Henson DB, Morris EJ (1993) Effect of uncorrected refractive errors upon central visual field testing. *Ophthalmic and Physiological Optics*, **13**: 339

Johnson CA, Adamo AJ, Lewis RA (1989) Evidence for a neural basis of age-related visual field loss in normal observers. *Investigative Ophthalmology*, **30**: 2056

Kanski J, McAllister J (1989). *Glaucoma: A Colour Manual of Diagnosis and Treatment.* London, Butterworths

Lindenmuth KA, Skuta GL, Rabbani R, Musch DC (1989) Effect of pupillary constriction on automated perimetry in normal eyes. *Ophthalmology*, **96**: 1289

Mikelberg FS, Drance SM, Schutzer M, Wijsman K (1987) The effect of miosis on visual field indices. *Documenta Ophthalmologica Proceedings Series*, **49**: 645

Miller NR, Newman NJ (1999) *Walsh and Hoyt's Clinical NeuroOphthalmology. The Essentials.* 5th edn. Baltimore, MD, Williams and Wilkins

Stamper R, Lieberman M, Drake M (1999). *Diagnosis and Therapy of the Glaucomas.* St Louis, Mosby

Further reading

Allergen Humphrey (1991) *Field Analyzer Owner's Manual*. San Leandro, CA, Humphrey Instruments (Carl Zeiss Group)

American Academy of Ophthalmology (1996) Automated perimetry. *Ophthalmology*, **103**: 1144

Anderson DR (1992) *Automated Static Perimetry*. St Louis, CV Mosby

Armaly MF (1969) Ocular pressure and visual fields. *Archives of Ophthalmology*, **81**: 25

Autzen T, Work K (1990) The effect of learning and age on short-term fluctuation and mean sensitivity of automated static perimetry. *Acta Ophthalmologica*, **68**: 327

Enoch JM (ed.) (1979) *Perimetric Standards and Perimetric Glossary of the International Council of Ophthalmology*. The Hague, W. Junck

Fankhauser F, Enoch JM (1962) The effect of blur on perimetric thresholds. *Archives of Ophthalmology*, **86**: 240

Gonzalez de la Rosa M, Pareja A (1997) Influence of the fatigue effect on the mean deviation measurement in perimetry. *European Journal of Ophthalmology*, **7**: 29

Haley MJ (1987) *The Field Analyzer Primer*, 2nd edn. San Leandro, CA, Humphrey Instruments

Herse PR (1992) Factors influencing normal perimetric thresholds. *Investigative Ophthalmology and Visual Science*, **33**: 611

Heuer DK, Anderson DR, Feuer WJ, Gressel MG (1987) The influence of refraction accuracy on automated perimetric threshold measurements. *Ophthalmology*, **94**: 1550

Hoyt WF, Tudor RC (1963) The course of papillary temporal retinal axons through the anterior optic nerve. A Nanta degeneration study in the primate. *Archives of Ophthalmology*, **69**: 503

Jaffe GJ, Alvarado JA, Juster RP (1986) Age-related changes of the normal visual field. *Archives of Ophthalmology*, **104**: 1021

Johnson C, Nelson-Quigg JM (1993) A prospective three year study of response properties of normal subjects and patients during automated perimetry. *Ophthalmology*, **100**: 269

Katz J, Sommer A, Witt K (1991) Reliability of visual field results over repeated testing. *Ophthalmology*, **98**: 70

Kline LB, Bajandas FJ (1995) *Neuro-Ophthalmology Review Manual*, 4th edn. Thorofare, NJ, Slack

Reitner A, Tittl M, Ergun E, Baradaran-Dilmaghani R (1996) The efficient use of perimetry for neuro-ophthalmic diagnosis. *British Journal of Ophthalmology*, **80**: 903

Rowe FJ (1998) Visual field analysis with Humphrey automated perimetry. Part I and II. *Eye News*, 4(6) 6–10; 5(1) 15–19

Rowe FJ (1999) *Idiopathic intracranial hypertension. Assessment of visual function and prognosis for visual outcome*. PhD thesis, APU Cambridge

Sarkies N (1987) Neurological visual fields. *British Orthoptic Journal*, **44**: 15

Taylor JF (ed.) (1995) *Medical Aspects of Fitness to Drive. A Guide for Medical Practitioners*. London, Medical Commission on Accident Prevention

Townsend JC, Selvin GJ, Griffin JR, Comer GW (1991) *Visual Fields – Clinical Case Presentations*. Boston, MA, Butterworth Heinemann

Weinreb RN, Perlman JP (1986) The effect of refractive correction on automated perimetric thresholds. *American Journal of Ophthalmology*, **101**: 706

Werner EB, Adelson A, Krupin T (1988) Effect of patient experience on the results of automated perimetry in clinically stable glaucoma patients. *Ophthalmology*, **95**: 764

Zalta AH (1989) Lens rim artefact in automated threshold perimetry. *Ophthalmology*, **96**: 1302

Chapter 2

Methods of visual field assessment

Visual field assessment may be manual or automated. Manual perimetry may use a kinetic and/or static technique, and perimeters include Goldmann perimetry, Friedmann perimetry and Bjerrum screens. Confrontation may be used during a patient's clinical examination as a very basic indication of the visual field. Automated perimetry predominantly uses a static technique, and perimeters include the Humphrey Field Analyser, Octopus perimeter, Dicon perimeter and Henson perimeter.

The Humphrey Automated Field Analyser and Goldmann manual perimeter method will be addressed specifically throughout this text for purposes of description and illustrations of visual field defects, as both of these perimeters are the methods most commonly employed for visual field assessment.

Presentation of visual field data

Data presentation may be in different forms.

(1) Map of isopters (Fig. 2.1). This is used to document the area of visual field and isopters are assessed with targets of differing size and luminance. This mode of presentation is used to display visual field results obtained with Goldmann perimetry.
(2) Luminance values (decibels; Fig. 2.2). Values are plotted at different points within the field of vision to give sensitivities at those points across the visual field. These decibel values are converted to a grey scale map and given statistical values when compared to age-matched normal results. This mode of presentation is used to display visual field results with Humphrey automated perimetry.

Goldmann manual perimeter

The Goldmann perimeter is a spherical projection perimeter (Colour Plate 2.1) which incorporates a system that allows direct registration of the target position.

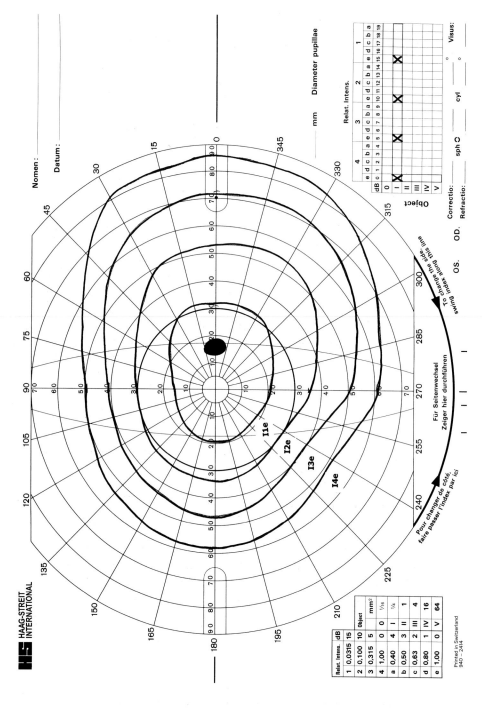

Figure 2.1 Map of isopters. The Goldmann chart shows the most commonly used target sizes and intensities.

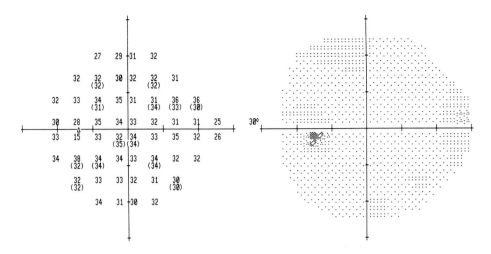

Figure 2.2 Luminance values (decibels). A plot is achieved of retinal sensitivity values in decibels.

The bowl has a radius of 30 cm and illumination of the bowl is constant and uniform. The target used to determine the boundaries and threshold of the visual field is projected onto the inside of the bowl. The target can be altered in size and luminous intensity, and both kinetic and static examination of the central and peripheral visual field can be achieved. There are six target sizes from the largest size V to the smallest size O (64, 16, 4, 1, $\frac{1}{4}$ and $\frac{1}{16}$ mm^2) with a difference of 5 decibels between each target size. Size O is generally not used as its results are inconsistent. There are two sets of grey filters to change the stimulus intensity (luminance). The first set includes four grey filters: 1.0, 0.315, 0.1 and 0.0315. The second set contains five grey filters: 1.0, 0.8, 0.63, 0.5 and 0.4. The filters change the target intensity in 1 decibel steps.

The bowl luminosity is set to 31.5 apostilb, which is the same as in Humphrey automated perimetry, and the brightness of the target is set to 1000 apostilb. These factors should be set by calibration and therefore provide a standardised examination at each test as the adaptive state of the eye is the same at each examination. The visual field can be compared over a variable time period in the knowledge that the examination conditions have remained constant. A V4e target calibrated at 1000 apostilb equates to 0 decibels.

The instrument is handled from the examiner's side and the fixation of the patient's eye can be constantly checked through a reticulated telescope. It is important to assess patient fixation continuously to ensure reliability of patient responses. The patient should be instructed to look continually towards the central fixation target. Both kinetic and static perimetry can be performed.

Kinetic perimetry

In kinetic perimetry a stimulus is moved from an area in which it is not seen (infrathreshold) into a region where it is visible (suprathreshold). The boundary between regions of invisibility and visibility is the isopter, a perimeter line that connects all points at which the stimulus has been seen. Kinetic quantitative perimetry uses a target of fixed size and brightness that is moved at a constant medium speed from the periphery into the visual field of the patient. This is undertaken in a number of different positions around the expected boundary of the visual field and an isopter plot is achieved. The position of the target in the sphere is clearly indicated on a large chart. This technique is repeated with targets of different size and brightness providing different suprathreshold isopters for the patient.

The horizontal and vertical meridians in particular should be assessed to detect visual field defects such as nasal steps and temporal sector defects. When assessing the peripheral visual field, a small bright target is normally used (I4e target is usually a sufficient size for the normal field). A small dim target is used for assessment of the central visual field (I2e target is usually a sufficient size for the normal field) and the patient's reading prescription must be used when testing the central field.

If the I2e target is unseen, the central field can be assessed with the I3e target. Where the peripheral field is constricted or if localised defects are noted, these can be further assessed with larger targets, commonly the III4e target and then further with the V4e target (largest brightest target). Driving fields for DVLA assessment should be undertaken with the III4e target size.

Movement of the target during perimetry should be approximately 2 degrees per second. The speed of movement is important. If moved too fast the target will travel quite a distance between being seen and responded to by the patient and being recorded by the perimetrist. This will have the effect of reducing the size and therefore the area of the visual field. If plotting an area of reduced visual field, this would appear larger than the actual size.

Static perimetry

Static quantitative perimetry may also be undertaken during which a target of known brightness at suprathreshold level is flashed on briefly within the plotted isopter boundaries of the patient's visual field. Static perimetry is mostly undertaken in the central 30 degrees and can be confined to areas known to be at risk in certain conditions, for example paracentral areas in optic disc disease and temporal field areas for temporal wedge or sector defects.

Procedures of examination using Goldmann perimetry were described by Armaly in 1969, and both kinetic boundaries and static responses of the visual field were tested. These procedures have been used for glaucoma monitoring. Modified testing strategies have been developed to test both kinetic and static boundaries (Fig. 2.3) and enable an accurate and repeatable assessment of the visual field while increasing the sensitivity of the testing strategy to detection of subtle visual field defects, particularly those of a scotomatous nature in which Humphrey perimetry has been proven to be superior at detection in the past.

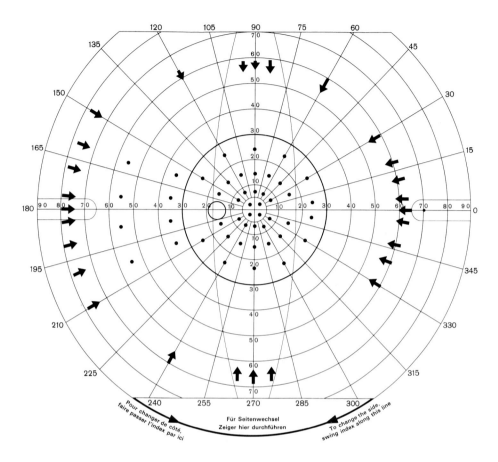

Figure 2.3 Goldmann assessment strategy. The arrows indicate kinetic perimetry locations and the points indicate static perimetry locations.

Patient set-up

The patient should be seated comfortably holding the response button in either hand. The button tip is usually pushed with the thumb; however, the patient may hold the button but press the tip against their leg. The patient should feel the click and hear the faint beep it makes.

The patient is instructed to look straight ahead at the central light. This target may be used for patients with visual acuity levels of 6/60 or better. If the patient has nystagmus but good fixation, they are asked to continue looking straight ahead towards the central target whilst observing their fixation through the telescope. In cases of poor visual acuity they are simply asked to keep looking in a straight ahead position.

The patient should wear an eye patch so that it completely occludes the non-tested eye. Their head should be placed squarely in the chin rest and against the forehead rest. An image of the patient's eye can be seen through the reticulated telescope of the perimeter, and the eye should be centred with the cross within the telescope by altering the chin rest position manually. Where trial frame lenses are used, these are placed before the tested eye as close to the eye as possible without touching the eyelashes.

When mapping the peripheral boundaries of the visual field, the patient is instructed to press the response button as soon as they are aware of a white light moving into their field of vision. When assessing static points, the patient is instructed to press the response button any time they are aware of a brief flash of white light, one at a time, outside central fixation during the test, of which some will appear bright and some dim.

Detection of visual field defect and detection of change

The Goldmann perimeter visual field assessment provides a mapping of peripheral and central sensitivities of the visual field result by plotting a variety of isopters relating to different target sizes and luminance intensities. To identify the presence of a visual field defect, it is imperative that the normal age matched perimeters and sensitivities of the visual field are known (see Fig. 2.1). A visual comparison can then be made by looking at both peripheral and central visual fields plotted by kinetic and static techniques.

Constriction of the visual field can be quantified in terms of extent of loss of visual field in degrees for a specific stimulus. Patterns of visual field loss can be identified, such as the presence of a quadrantanopia, scotoma or arcuate visual field defect. As always, a comparison of the visual field results from either eye is essential.

A comparison of visual field results may be made to detect any change in visual field status over time. To achieve a comparison it is important that the same target sizes and luminance intensities are used at retesting, so that a direct comparison of 'like with like' is achieved. Change in size of isopter or extent of localised visual field loss, e.g. scotoma size, can easily be identified in the knowledge that the visual field results have been obtained under repeatable testing conditions.

Humphrey automated perimeter

The Humphrey automated perimeter is a sensitive and highly precise assessor of visual field. It is a single unit, fully automatic, computerised, projection perimeter (Colour Plate 2.2). The background illumination is 31.5 apostilb which is set as a standard by the International Perimetric Society and is the same as for Goldmann perimetry. The Humphrey automated perimeter uses stimuli that are projected onto the bowl area and which are varied in luminosity over a range of 51 decibels. The stimulus size can be varied, but not during a test. The size is set before the test programme is run (Heijl & Patella 2002). A Goldmann size III target is usually used which is considered small enough to detect small scotomas but large enough to be relatively unaffected by residual refractive errors (Sloan 1961).

Screening programmes

Screening programmes involve the use of suprathreshold tests where the visual field is assessed using targets of brightness level above that which would be expected to be seen for the age of the patient. They determine the threshold level for one point in each quadrant of the visual field and adjust these values to provide a central reference level which is the brightness level at which the test is run. Each point is then screened at 6 decibels brighter than the expected threshold at that point. The stimuli are thus brighter in the periphery and dimmer in the centre (Heijl & Patella 2002).

In a 'threshold related strategy', if the stimulus is seen, this is registered. If unseen it is retested at the same intensity, and if still unseen is registered as a miss. In a 'three zone strategy', if a point is not seen on two occasions at this level, it is later retested at 0 decibels and if seen is recorded as a relative defect; if unseen, it is recorded as an absolute defect. However, there is no information provided as to the extent of the visual field defect in regard to the depth of visual field loss. This is achieved with threshold assessment. In a 'quantify defects strategy', all missed points are thresholded. The area of visual field defect can be plotted and expansion of this area over time with progression can be seen.

Threshold programmes

Threshold tests provide more detailed information than suprathreshold tests. Detection of visual field loss is aided by comparison of the test result with that of a normal standard. A series of suprathreshold tests will demonstrate expansion of the area of involvement of field loss. However, threshold tests demonstrate deepening of the area of visual loss in addition to the expansion of this area (Heijl & Patella 2002).

During each test, the computer presents stimuli randomly at each of the set testing points of the programme. The most commonly used programmes are the 24-2 and 30-2 threshold programmes. The 24 degree strategy tests 54 points; the 24-2 programme has a 6 degree spaced grid offset from the vertical and horizontal meridia. The 30 degree strategy tests 76 points; this programme also has a 6 degree spaced grid offset from the vertical and horizontal meridia.

A stair step or bracketing process is used. Initially four points are tested in order to determine the threshold level at those points; these are then used as a starting level for neighbouring points, and so on until the entire visual field has been completed. Points are tested twice where the anticipated response is outside 5 decibels of that expected, and the second response obtained is bracketed on the final printout of results.

For **full threshold testing**, the stimulus intensity is increased in 4 decibel steps until recorded; it is then decreased to below the threshold level and increased again until recorded, in 2 decibel steps, to confirm the threshold level at that point. A **full from prior** strategy may also be used in which the last test to be performed is recalled and the threshold levels for each point from the last test used as starting levels for the current test. The stimuli are initially started at a level 2 decibels higher than the previous threshold and the test then continues as for a full threshold programme. The **fastpac** strategy for threshold testing determines threshold sensitivity in 3 decibel steps only, thus speeding up the test process. This enables the patient to finish the test more quickly, an advantage where patient fatigue or illness is a problem. The **SITA** (Swedish Interactive Thresholding Algorithm) also uses full threshold and fastpac testing, but is a faster method of assessing the visual field because of its interactive nature with patient responses and speed. SITA is available on the Series 7 perimeter models. **SITA standard** has a testing programme of 4 and 2 decibel steps similar to the full threshold programme. **SITA fast** has a testing programme of 3 decibel steps. SITA standard has been proven to provide as accurate and reliable field results as with normal full threshold fields, and therefore can be recommended for routine visual field assessment (Wild *et al.* 1999).

SITA considers many factors in determining what stimuli to present at each point during the test. These factors include age, normative data, detailed characteristics of abnormal and normal tests, and patient responses so far in the test. They are combined and weighted into the SITA visual field model which continually produces updated calculations of the threshold at each point. The SITA standard programme takes half the time of the standard full threshold programme and is considered more accurate and reproducible (Bengtsson & Heijl 1998; Bengtsson *et al.* 1998). The SITA fast programme takes half the time of the fastpac programme but with similar accuracy and reproducibility.

The SITA algorithm is based on four separate investigative computer applications which all interact with each other: (1) smart questions which determine the choice of stimulus brightness throughout the examination dependent on patient responses during the test; (2) smart pacing which determines the reaction times of the patient to the stimuli presented and adjusts presentation accordingly; (3) knowledge of when to terminate the examination, which allows the termination of the examination once a required number of stimulus presentations has been achieved at the given stimuli locations (this allows the instrument to spend extra time at locations requiring additional information and less time at locations where the responses are highly consistent); (4) post-examination process which allows processing of information not from individual threshold points, but from neighbouring points also, together with interpretation of patient reliability (Heijl & Patella 2002).

Patient set-up

The patient should be seated comfortably, holding the response button in either hand. The button tip is usually pushed with the thumb; however, if the patient has difficulty holding the button (due to arthritis for example), they may hold the button but press the tip against their leg. The patient should feel the click and hear the faint beep it makes. If the patient holds the button down for a period of time, the test will pause until it is released.

The patient is instructed to look straight ahead at the central light. In cases of poor visual acuity they may be asked to look towards the centre of the four lights positioned just below the central light.

The patient should wear an eye patch so that it completely occludes the non-tested eye. Their head should be placed squarely in the chin rest and against the forehead rest. An image of the patient's eye can be seen on the monitor; the eye should be centred with the cross within the monitor by altering the chin rest position with the horizontal and vertical alignment wheels. Where trial frame lenses are used, these are placed before the tested eye as close to the eye as possible without touching the eyelashes.

Other lights will flash, one at a time, off centre during the test, some bright and some dim. The patient is instructed to press the button each time one of these lights is seen. The best time for the patient to blink is as they press the button.

Reliability indices

Test reliability is monitored by determination of fixation losses, false positive and false negative responses. As with all perimetry tests, it is important to monitor patient fixation. Patient fixation can be monitored visually during the test, but there is an in-built assessment of fixation which is achieved by the test programme periodically presenting stimuli in the patient's blind spot area (Heijl & Karkau 1977). The patient's blind spot is initially localised (usually between 10 to 20 degrees along the horizontal meridian in the temporal visual field) and during the testing procedure, approximately 10% of the stimuli are presented in the blind spot. The number of times the patient responds to seeing this light is recorded. If the patient is maintaining steady fixation, there should be no response to the stimulus in the blind spot area. However, should their fixation change due to movement of their head or with wandering eye movements, a response will be made to this stimuli and this will be recorded as a **fixation loss**.

In addition to monitoring fixation losses, the 7 series perimeter models include **gaze tracking** which is a measure of gaze direction each time a stimulus is presented. Lines with an upward direction represent gaze error at each stimulus presentation. A full measure indicates a gaze error of 10 degrees of more. Lines with a downward direction represent an inability of the perimeter to measure gaze direction at that stimulus presentation (Heijl & Patella 2002).

During the test, the machine will at times move the projection device but will not present a stimulus. Should the patient respond despite the absence of a stimulus, this is recorded as a **false positive**. A high false positive score is often seen in 'trigger happy' patients who press the response button frequently despite not seeing stimuli. These patients also continue to respond to actual stimuli, with the result that stimuli are presented at these points at consecutively higher sensitivities. Abnormally high sensitivity decibel values are thus achieved (see Chapter 13). SITA programmes estimate the rate of false positive catch trials by determining the number of responses that fall outside the normal response time (Wild 1997).

Throughout the test, the machine also projects a stimulus at a point which has already had a positive response to a certain decibel value. The patient should therefore respond to this. However, if there is no response, this is recorded as a **false negative**. False negatives may be seen in patients with poor reliability, but also in those with early onset of visual loss or changing visual field status as there may be relative scotomas and visual response in this area may vary (Bengtsson & Heijl 2000). False negatives may also be a sign of fatigue; allowing the patient a break during the test may alleviate this problem. Where fixation losses, false positive or false negative responses are recorded as exceeding 33% of stimuli, this will be documented as low patient reliability on the printout of results.

Interpretation

The statistical package produces an in depth statistical analysis of the visual field test results. It performs three important functions:

(1) It can point out suspicious areas that otherwise might not be evident until subsequent testing
(2) It can identify areas that look suspicious but which, in fact, compare favourably with normal data
(3) Using results from a series of tests, it can provide a highly sensitive and informative analysis of changes in the patient's visual field over time.

The Humphrey perimeter computer contains information of the decibel values expected at each point of the normal age matched visual field over a wide age range. **Statpac** is the statistical programme used to analyse the data from single, or multiple, visual field assessments using threshold programmes. Once a test has finished, the results of that test are then compared to the computer's database of age matched normals to determine whether the test result is also normal or whether a visual field defect has been recorded.

A **glaucoma hemifield test** is performed as part of the analysis of results. This compares areas of the superior visual field with corresponding areas of the inferior visual field (Fig. 2.4) to determine whether the response to stimuli is comparable in the superior and inferior areas of the visual field. Where there is localised visual field deficit, a difference will be documented and a borderline, or outside normal limits, response will be obtained for the hemifield.

Global indices are provided on the visual field printouts and include the mean deviation (MD), pattern standard deviation (PSD), short term fluctuation (SF) and corrected pattern standard deviation (CPSD) (Fig. 2.5).

The **mean deviation** is the overall departure of the average deviation of the visual field result from that expected of a normal field of the same age group. In normal results this value is low, and in abnormal visual field results the value is high. The mean deviation is derived from the numbers in the total deviation plot. It is the weighted mean of all the numbers displayed in the total deviation plot which are the deviations from the average normal values for age. All tested locations are included except for the two which might include the physiological blind spot. Each deviation from normal is weighted according to the variance of normal values at that location; thus points with low variance (closer to fixation) are more important than points with higher variance (larger range of normal). The mean deviation index signifies overall severity of visual field loss. It is affected both by the degree of loss and the number of affected locations. If the mean deviation is lower than found in 10% of the normal population with reliable visual fields, a percentile is given at five significant levels ($p < 10\%$, 5%, 2%, 1% and 0.5%).

The **pattern standard deviation** is determined by the variation from the normal hill of vision. The normal curve of a visual field has the highest decibel value at the

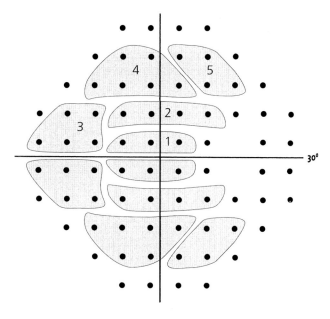

Figure 2.4 Glaucoma hemifield test location of comparative areas. Pattern deviation probability scores in five zones of the superior field are compared to corresponding zones in the inferior field. Reproduced with permission (Heijl 2002).

central foveal area, with gradual reduction towards the periphery; there should be no response at the blind spot. A normal hill of vision will give a low pattern standard deviation value. Where there is localised loss of vision, such as with paracentral scotomas or arcuate defects, the hill of vision will be deviated from the norm and a high pattern standard deviation value will be obtained. As more visual field becomes involved with pathology, with overall reduction in sensitivity, the pattern standard deviation value will change to a lower value as the overall hill of vision achieves an equilibrium across all areas of the visual field.

Short term fluctuation is monitored throughout the test. Ten pre-selected points are checked twice to determine reliability of response. The ten locations that are pre-selected may be an unrepresentative sample of stimulus locations and may not include damaged areas of the visual field (Casson *et al.* 1990); the value may therefore not always be representative of the status of the visual field. Where both values at one point are equivalent or within 4 decibels of each other, this is taken as a reliable response. However, where values at one point are greater than 5 decibels in difference, reliability at this point is questionable. This may be due to poor fixation or lack of concentration, but occasionally may be due to early or progressive visual field loss which also results in false negative responses. Short term fluctuation values are usually between 1 and 2.5 decibels in a normal visual field result.

The **corrected pattern standard deviation** takes into consideration any intratest variability as noted by the short term fluctuation. This will highlight any suspicious points which, although they may be within normal decibel values for that point, may indicate the early onset of visual deficit and therefore should be observed for possible progression. The corrected pattern standard deviation will return to lower

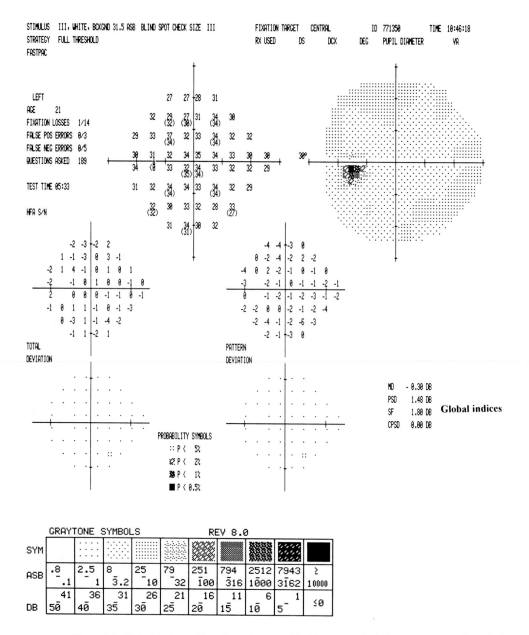

Figure 2.5 Global indices. Note the values provided for mean deviation, pattern standard deviation, short-term fluctuation and corrected pattern standard deviation.

values as visual field loss increases in severity. When the entire field of vision becomes involved, the hill of vision is then depressed as a whole.

Where the mean deviation, pattern standard deviation or corrected pattern standard deviation values exceed those found in 10% of the normal population data, a percentage is given at five significance levels (10%, 5%, 2%, 1% and 0.5%).

A number of different printouts of the test results may be obtained. The **three in one** printout (Fig. 2.6) provides a greyscale, a defect depth grid and a numeric grid. The greyscale gives an immediate view of the visual field, and the scale at the bottom of the chart shows the corresponding values of the greyscale in apostilbs and decibels. Each change in the greyscale tone is equivalent to a 5 decibel change in threshold. However, as a result of the grid spacing, small defects can be missed when interpreting the result without reference to other information provided in the printout. The numeric grid gives the patient responses at each point in decibel values. Points which are at least 5 decibels less than expected are checked a second time and the value shown in parentheses represents the threshold found on the second check. The defect grid shows the difference of the patient responses to those expected from a normal visual field.

A **single field analysis** (Fig. 2.7) provides six field plots, a greyscale, a numeric grid plus a total deviation grid and pattern standard deviation grid with their relevant probability plots. The total deviation is the deviation from normal values and its probability plot shows the associated probability value for each point and its variation from the norm. Probability values are represented as percentages of 5%, 2%, 1% or 0.5%. These values represent the likelihood of a defect occurring 'by chance' and as a result indicate the significance of such a defect. The pattern deviation is similar to the total deviation; however, it adjusts the field according to any overall depression, such as that which occurs with cataracts. It will also adjust the field if the overall sensitivity is high for the visual field; this has the advantage that localised areas of visual loss which may have been obscured by an overall elevation or depression in sensitivity of the visual field will be highlighted in the pattern deviation. A probability plot again provides the associated values for each point and their variation from the norm. The glaucoma hemifield test value represents a comparison of the mirror images of the superior and inferior visual fields in order to detect any significant difference in the threshold values of each half of the visual field, for example as would be found in arcuate defects. Visual field defects of varying conditions are thus easily identified from single field analysis.

Where a patient has been assessed on more than one occasion, the visual fields can be compared from one visit to the next. **Overview** printouts (Fig. 2.8) present each visual field in succession, with the greyscale, total deviation and probability plots for the total and pattern deviations; the global indices are also included. From this, a comparison can be made visually of the presence of progression of visual loss.

Change analysis (Fig. 2.9) will give a statistical evaluation of change in visual field over time. Global indices are summarised in chronological order and dashed reference lines indicate the $p < 5\%$ and $p < 1\%$ limits for the normal population. A box plot is used to graphically illustrate the visual field responses. The entire box plot from tail to tail represents the entire visual field responses. The heights of the various portions of the box plot indicate the degrees to which different points are more severely affected than others or the variability in the amount of involvement of the various points. The lower and upper tails each represent 15% of points, and the centre box represents 70%. The lower tail represents the worst points (lowest decibel values) and the upper tail represents the best points (highest decibel values). The normal box plot is shown to the left side of the table. Where there is

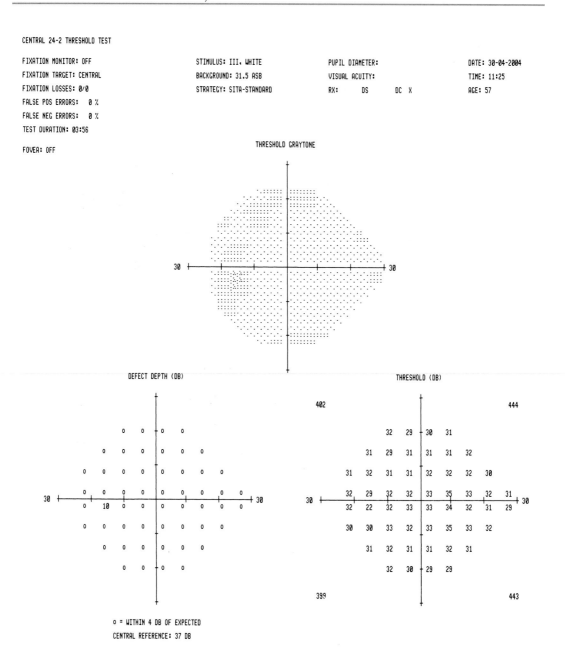

Figure 2.6 Three in one printout. Greyscale, defect depth grid and numeric grid (decibel values) are provided.

localised visual field loss affecting no more than 15% of the field, only the lower tail will appear elongated, demonstrating depression of the visual field for those points. Where there is complete constriction and involvement of the entire visual field, the whole box plot will be depressed on the table. When a series of these boxes are plotted for a succession of visual fields, the change in the character of the field over

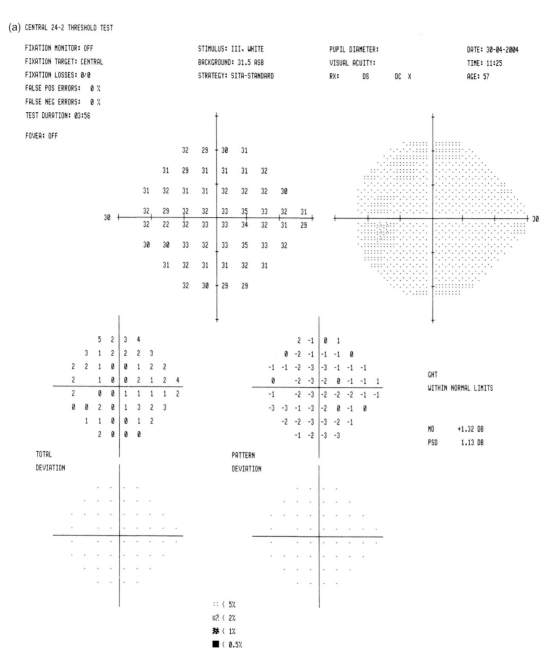

Figure 2.7 Single field analysis printout. Greyscale, numeric grid, total deviation grid, pattern standard deviation grid and probability plots for the latter two grids are provided. (a) Normal result: there are no deficits on the probability plots and the glaucoma hemifield test is normal. (b) Abnormal result: there are defects present on the probability plots with values of *p* < 0.5%. The glaucoma hemifield test is outside normal limits.

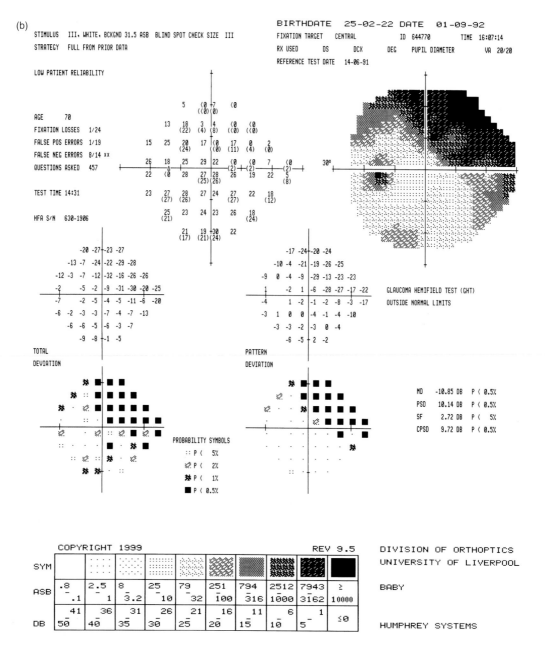

Figure 2.7 (Continued)

time can be noted, e.g. a short box that remains the same size but moves progressively downwards over time represents progressive generalised depression without local defects. Lengthening of the box, especially the inferior arm, over time indicates the development and deepening of localised defects. A long box on the initial examination that stays the same length and moves downwards is caused by a progressive

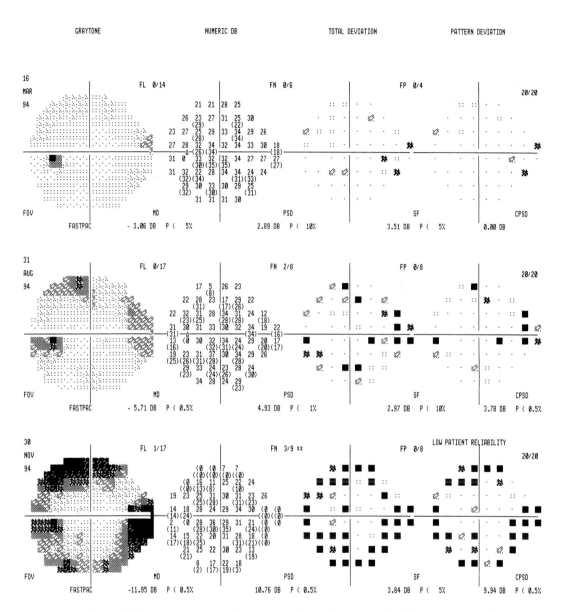

Figure 2.8 Overview printout. Greyscale, total deviation grid, probability plots for total deviation and pattern standard deviation grids and global indices values are provided. In this abnormal result note the progression of visual field loss from very minimal involvement (reduced nasal sensitivity) to development of superior and inferior arcuate visual field defects.

generalised depression superimposed on a localised defect (Rowe 1998). Progression of any defect is therefore quickly recognised from change analysis printouts.

Linear regression analysis will be performed where there are more than five visual fields. Where progression of visual field loss is deemed significant, the message 'mean deviation slope significant' will appear. The linear regression analysis tests the hypothesis that there is no change in the visual field (the slope is 0). If this is rejected at the $p < 5\%$ level or less, the slope is significant.

Further analysis of glaucoma visual fields may be obtained with the **glaucoma change probability** analysis (Fig. 2.10). The first and second visual field results are combined as an average and consecutive fields are then compared to this for progression of the condition. Where it is not possible to obtain an average of the first and second visual fields because of insufficient data, the first field only is used for comparison. The printout provides a greyscale of the current test, the total deviation plot, the change from the average baseline plot and its associated probability plot. Point by point analysis is documented on the probability plot where solid triangles represent significant deterioration of the visual field and open triangles represent areas of improvement.

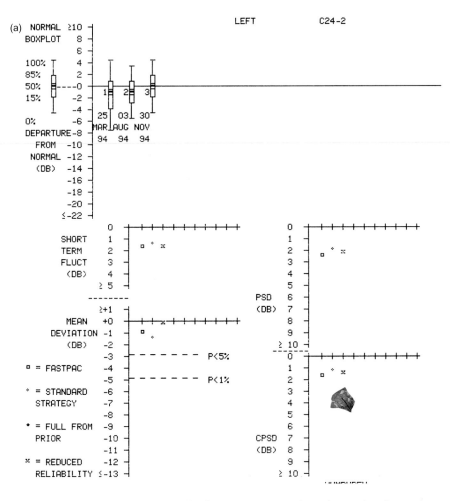

Figure 2.9 Change analysis printout. Boxplot, linear regression analysis (if more than five results compared) and global indices values are provided. (a) Normal result: the box plot remains central and global indices are within normal limits. (b) Abnormal result: there is an increase in boxplot size with the lower tail at −22 decibels. There are decreasing plots for the global indices with values at $p < 1\%$.

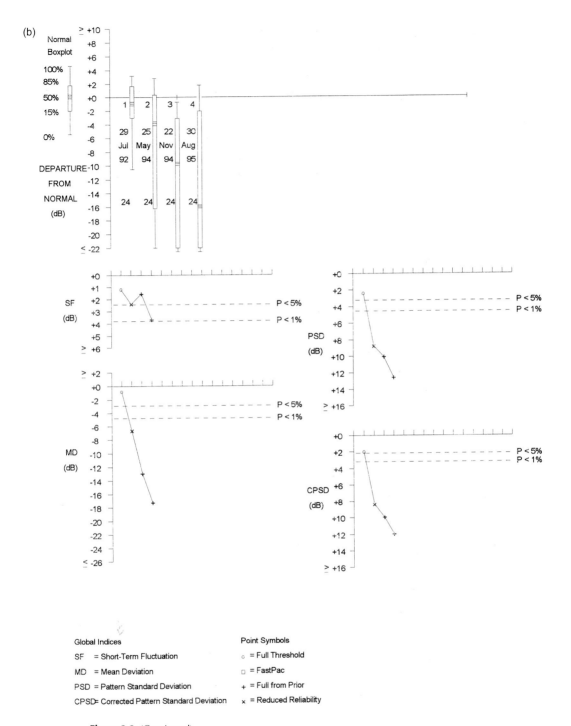

Figure 2.9 (Continued)

Detection of visual field defect and detection of change

Diagnostic accuracy depends not only on the selection of the correct programme, the quality of the test procedure and the technical administration, but also on the criteria used to judge abnormality or progression and the judgement used to correlate test results with the other clinical information. The outcome of a given examination is affected by a number of factors. Such factors determine the absolute value of sensitivity at a given location and also the variability in response at that location, both within a single visual field examination (short-term fluctuation) and between examinations (long-term fluctuation) and can limit the usefulness of automated perimetry for the evaluation of visual field progression (O'Brien & Wild 1995).

Progression is frequently deemed to have occurred only by retrospective examination of a large series of visual field plots. Some factors can be controlled by the clinician, such as pupil size and the correction of refractive error, but other factors may be difficult to eliminate. Some evidence as to the quality of the patient performance is given by the reply to the catch trials which assess the number of fixation losses and the number of false positive and false negative responses. A relatively low

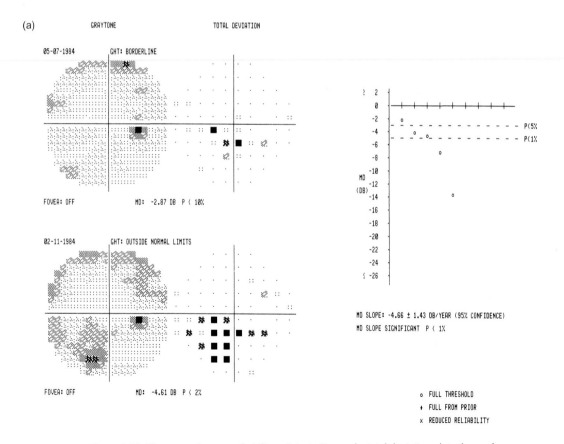

Figure 2.10 Glaucoma change probability printout. Greyscale, total deviation plot, change from average baseline plot and probability plot are provided.

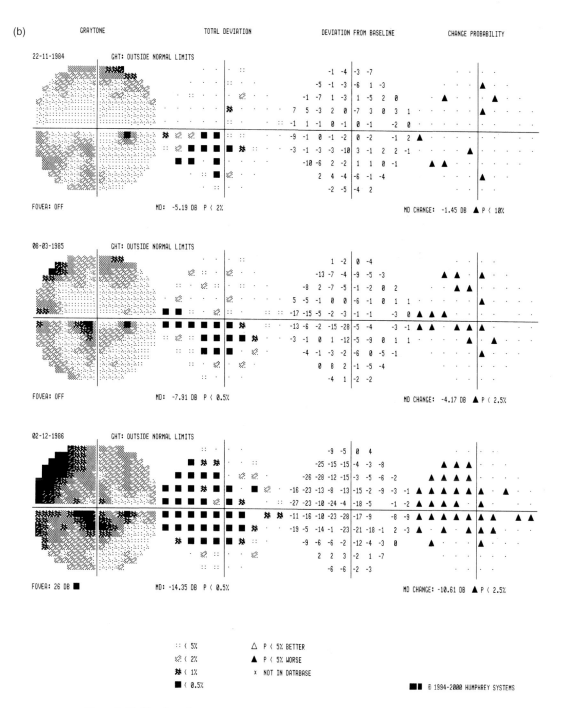

Figure 2.10 (Continued)

number of unreliable tests have been reported for both initial and follow up visits, and the majority of unreliable visual field tests are sporadic events. As a result, it has been concluded that automated perimetry can provide a reliable means of following patients over extended periods of time (Johnson & Nelson-Quigg 1993).

Single field analysis, overview and change analysis are of considerable value for the complete interpretation of visual field results. The presence of a visual field abnormality will be quite obvious in many patients, for example, the presence of a homonymous hemianopia in a patient with a known recent stroke/cerebrovascular accident. The difficulty arises with assessing visual fields for abnormalities that are not obvious, such as subtle changes that occur in early glaucoma. A visual field must first be assessed for its reliability, looking at factors such as fixation stability, false positive responses and false negative responses. The pattern deviation plot will give the statistical value of each point of the visual field test compared to age matched normal values. A localised visual field defect can be determined where the pattern deviation plot shows a cluster of three or more non-edge points at a $p < 5\%$ level (i.e. these points have sensitivities that occur in fewer than 5% of the normal population and are therefore considered a significant departure from the norm) and one of the points is at a $p < 1\%$ level (i.e. sensitivity that occurs in fewer than 1% of the normal population). This cluster of points should also be found in an area associated with the deficits that most commonly occur in the ocular disease suspected; for example, within the nerve fibre bundle for conditions such as glaucoma or optic disc swelling (Rowe 1998). The corrected pattern standard deviation will adjust for general sensitivity changes occurring across the visual field; values of less than 5% on this chart are confirmation of the likelihood that a visual field abnormality does actually exist. A comparison of the superior visual field to the inferior visual field is also of benefit in detecting abnormalities within cluster areas using the glaucoma hemifield test (Heijl & Patella 2002).

Major change in visual field status will be recognised easily, as severe deterioration or vast improvements in visual field loss are not likely to be due to long-term fluctuations. Minor changes may be due to short-term or long-term fluctuations; therefore slight progression can be ascertained only by determining that a number of points have altered by an amount that would not occur frequently in stable or normal visual fields and are at a level of $p < 5\%$ or $p < 1\%$.

Detection of change in visual fields can be difficult, particularly when considering the presence of normal physiological fluctuation that occurs not only during the test but also over a period of time from test to test. There is also the aspect of the learning curve that should be considered, particularly for early initial visual field assessments.

It is important to detect a change in visual field results that occurs due to disease rather than to a normal physiological variation in performance on visual field testing. Short- and long-term fluctuations will occur in both normal and abnormal visual fields; sensitivity can alter by 1–2 decibels across the normal visual field. Therefore change in visual field result due to ocular disease must exceed that which might occur purely due to normal variations of the visual field during the test and/or over time.

The change analysis printout is of value when examining fields for progression of visual field loss. It provides an analytical summary of changes in visual field over a period of time (Heijl & Patella 2002). The change analysis also provides a plot of global indices, including mean deviation values. The global indices are summarised in chronological order and dashed reference lines indicate the $p < 5\%$ and $p < 1\%$ limits for the normal population. When assessing visual fields for progression, all global indices are considered in relation to each other. With visual field progression, the short term fluctuation value usually increases due to variability at abnormal points and may then decrease when the field worsens further. The pattern standard deviation and corrected pattern standard deviation also rise as visual field loss initially develops, but then decrease as more of the field becomes involved (Pearson *et al.* 1990). However, the mean deviation index deteriorates progressively as the visual field worsens.

A plot of the mean deviation over time is helpful in the assessment of visual field progression; it does not give as complete an exposition of the visual field data as the box plot, for example, but it does permit a statistical test to be done to see if any trend towards deterioration is real or could be simply a result of test variability. The mean deviation index deteriorates progressively as the visual field worsens, but it may change slowly. For the plot of the mean deviation over a series of examinations, there is a regression analysis of mean deviation values over time which approximately takes into account the time of the examination, not simply its sequential number. If at least five visual fields are available, regression analysis will be performed indicating if there is a statistically significant change over time. In such cases the slope (decibels per year) and degree of statistical significance will be given; if the slope is negative and statistically significant, it indicates that the deterioration is not likely to be just a chance finding based on measurement variability.

Humphrey Field Analyzer machines can offer different threshold algorithms for designated programmes and a change in algorithm from test to test may influence sensitivity estimates so that the visual field result appears better or worse on subsequent testing. The SITA standard programme produces thresholds higher than full threshold analysis (Bengtsson & Heijl 1998) and as such the visual field result may appear similar if the programme has been switched from full threshold to SITA standard for subsequent testing. Early signs of progression may therefore be masked (Spry *et al.* 2001).

Stato-kinetic dissociation

Defects present on automated perimetry tend to be more extensive compared with those present on manual perimetry (Beck *et al.* 1985; Wall & George 1987; Wedemeyer *et al.* 1989). This is likely to be related to threshold static perimetry being more sensitive than kinetic perimetry combined with suprathreshold static testing. This can be explained by two factors. A moving stimulus is more visible than a non-moving one, and this may be more evident in defective regions of the visual field. This is known as the Riddoch phenomenon or stato-kinetic dissociation. It is therefore easier to see a Goldmann target. Humphrey perimetry gives a briefer flash of light stimulus compared to the Goldmann stimulus. It is therefore more difficult to see the Humphrey stimuli (Hudson & Wild 1992). The duration of a stimulus is important for a brief flash (e.g. $\frac{1}{100}$ s versus $\frac{2}{100}$ s) but duration does not change the visibility of a stimulus after a certain critical time (approximately $\frac{1}{3}$

s or longer). After this length of time, duration does not matter because maximum temporal summation has occurred.

References

Armaly MF (1969) Ocular pressure and visual fields. *Archives of Ophthalmology*, **81**: 25

Beck RW, Bergstrom TJ, Lichter PR (1985) A clinical comparison of visual field testing with a new automated perimeter (Humphrey) and the Goldmann perimeter. *Ophthalmology*, **92**: 77

Bengtsson B, Heijl A (1998) SITA Fast, a new rapid perimetric threshold test. Description of methods and evaluation in patients with manifest and suspect glaucoma. *Acta Ophthalmologica Scandinavica*, **76**: 431

Bengtsson B, Heijl A (2000) False-negative responses in glaucoma perimetry: indicators of patient performance or test reliability. *Investigative Ophthalmology and Vision Science*, **41**: 2201

Bengtsson B, Heijl A, Olsson J (1998) Evaluation of a new threshold visual field strategy, SITA, in normal subjects. *Acta Ophthalmologica Scandinavica*, **76**: 165

Casson E, Shapiro L, Johnson C (1990) Short-term fluctuation as an estimate of variability in visual field data. *Investigative Ophthalmology and Vision Science*, **31**: 2459

Heijl A, Krakau C (1977) A note on fixation during perimetry. *Acta Ophthalmologica*, **55**: 854

Heijl A, Patella VM (2002) *The Field Analyzer Primer. Essential Perimetry*, 3rd edn. Dublin, CA, Carl Zeiss Meditec

Hudson C, Wild JM (1992) Assessment of physiologic statokinetic dissociation by automated perimetry. *Investigative Ophthalmology and Visual Science*, **33**: 3162

Johnson CA, Nelson-Quigg JM (1993) A prospective 3-year study of response properties of normal subjects and patients during automated perimetry. *Ophthalmology*, **100**: 269

O'Brien C, Wild JM (1995) Automated perimetry in glaucoma – room for improvement? *British Journal of Ophthalmology*, **79**: 200

Pearson PA, Baldwin LB, Smith TJ (1990) The relationship of mean defect to corrected loss variance in glaucoma and ocular hypertension. *Ophthalmologica*, **200**: 16

Rowe FJ (1998) Visual field analysis with Humphrey automated perimetry. Parts I and II. *Eye News*, **4**(6): 6–10; 5(1): 15–19

Sloan L (1961) Area and luminance of test object as variables in examination of the visual field by projection perimetry. *Vision Research*, **1**: 121

Spry P, Johnson C, Mckendrick A, Turpin A (2001) Variability of components of standard automated perimetry and frequency-doubling technology perimetry. *Investigative Ophthalmology and Vision Science*, **42**: 1404

Wall M, George DN (1987) Visual loss in pseudotumor cerebri. *Archives of Neurology*, **44**: 170

Wedemeyer L, Keltner JL, Johnson CA (1989) Statokinetic dissociation in optic nerve disease. *Documenta Ophthalmologica Proceedings Series*, **43**: 9

Wild JM (1997) SITA – A new outlook for visual field examination for primary and shared care. *Optician*, **213**: 212

Wild JM, Pacey I, Hancock S, Cunliffe I (1999) Between-algorithm, between-individual differences in normal perimetric sensitivity: full threshold FASTPAC and SITA. Swedish Interactive Threshold Algorithm. *Investigative Ophthalmology and Visual Science*, **40**: 1152

Further reading

Anderson DR (1992) *Automated Static Perimetry*. St Louis, CV Mosby

Asman P, Heijl A (1992) Glaucoma hemifield test. Automated visual field evaluation. *Archives of Ophthalmology*, **110**: 812

Bengtsson B, Heijl A (1998) Evaluation of a new perimetric threshold strategy, SITA, in patients with manifest and suspect glaucoma. *Acta Ophthalmologica Scandinavica*, **76**: 268

Bengtsson B, Olsson J, Heijl A, Rootzen H (1997) A new generation of algorithms for computerized threshold perimetry, SITA. *Acta Ophthalmologica*, **75**: 368

Bengtsson B (2000) Reliability of computerized perimetric threshold tests as assessed by reliability indices and threshold reproducibility in patients with suspect and manifest glaucoma. *Acta Ophthalmologica*, **78**: 519

Birch MK, Wishart PK, O'Donnell NP (1995) Determining progressive visual field loss in serial Humphrey visual fields. *Ophthalmology*, **102**: 1227

Enoch JM (ed.) (1979) *Perimetric Standards and Perimetric Glossary of the International Council of Ophthalmology*. The Hague, W. Junck

Flamer J, Drance S, Schulzer M (1983) The estimation and testing of the components of long-term fluctuation of the differential light threshold. *Documents Ophthalmology Proceedings Series*, **35**: 383

Johnson CA, Keltner JL (1987) Optimal rates of movement for kinetic perimetry. *Archives of Ophthalmology*, **105**: 73

Rowe FJ (1999) *Idiopathic intracranial hypertension. Assessment of visual function and prognosis for visual outcome*. PhD thesis, APU Cambridge

Chapter 3

Programme choice

An advantage of visual field assessment is that it provides a representation of the visual field integrity, i.e. integrity of the neural pathway throughout the extent of the visual pathway from the eye to the visual cortex. The visual field assessment plots the central and/or peripheral field of vision. Repeated measures aid detection of change in visual status and aid differential diagnosis of conditions.

Choice of perimeter

There are a variety of programmes that may be chosen for field assessment, dependent on the ocular condition. Peripheral field programmes are available with Humphrey automated perimetry but Goldmann perimetry can be recommended for detailed evaluation of the peripheral field boundaries by an experienced perimetrist. Goldmann perimetry is also recommended for assessment of the blind spot area. Patients with poor fixation may find Goldmann perimetry easier to achieve than Humphrey perimetry, and those patients with poor vision are more likely to have a reliable field plotted on Goldmann perimetry with a V4e target whereas a minimal or no field would be plotted on the Humphrey perimeter. Table 3.1 provides some general indications for choice of perimeter.

Humphrey automated perimeter

Humphrey screening programmes

Version 6 series (Colour Plate 3.1)

Glaucoma	Armaly central, Armaly full field, nasal step.
Central 30 degree tests	Central 40, central 76, central 80, central 166 (these refer to the number of points tested).
Peripheral	Full field 81, full field 120, full field 246, peripheral 68 (Fig. 3.1).
Custom tests	Custom tests allow you to test just a few points, or to add further points to an existing strategy.

Table 3.1 Choice of perimeter: general indications.

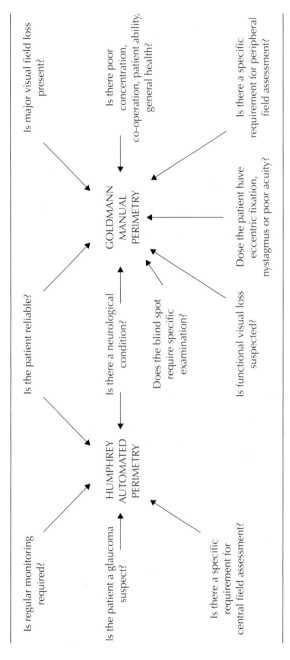

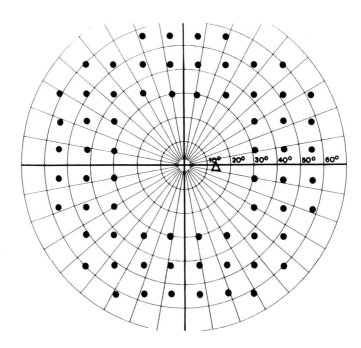

Figure 3.1 Peripheral 68 strategy. Each division on the horizontal and vertical meridia of the visual field printout represents 10 degrees. Reproduced with permission (Haley 1987).

Version 7 series (see Colour Plate 2.2)

Glaucoma	Nasal step, central Armaly screening, full field Armaly.
Central 30 degree tests	Central 40, central 64, central 76 and central 80.
Peripheral	Full field 81, full field 120, full field 135 and full field 246, peripheral 60.

Humphrey threshold programmes

Version 6 series

Central	24-1, 24-2 (Fig. 3.2), 30-1, 30-2 (Fig. 3.3).
Peripheral	60-1, 60-4 (Fig. 3.1), nasal step, temporal crescent.
Speciality	Neurological 20 or 50, central 10-2 (Fig. 3.4), macula (Fig. 3.5).
Custom tests	

Version 7 series

Central	24-2 (Fig. 3.2), 30-2 (Fig. 3.3).
Peripheral	60-2, nasal step.
Speciality	10-2 (Fig. 3.4), macula (Fig. 3.5).

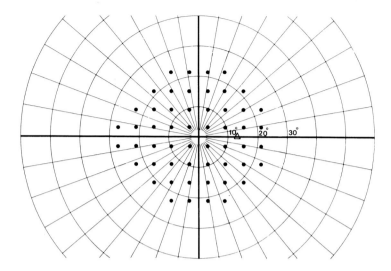

Figure 3.2 24-2 strategy. Each division on the horizontal and vertical meridia of the visual field printout represents 10 degrees. Reproduced with permission (Haley 1987).

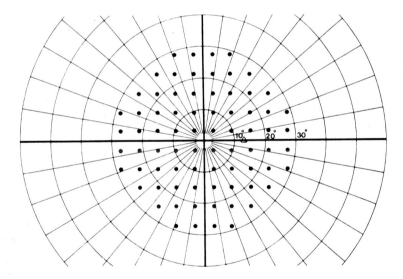

Figure 3.3 30-2 strategy. Each division on the horizontal and vertical meridia of the visual field printout represents 10 degrees. Reproduced with permission (Haley 1987).

Central test stimuli are spaced 6 degrees apart, whilst peripheral test stimuli are spaced 12 degrees apart (Heijl & Patella 2002). The majority of optic nerve fibres transmit information from the central visual field; 60–70% of optic nerve fibres subserve the central 30 degrees. It is therefore in the central field that subtle and early lesions can be found. It should be remembered that some of the screening tests take more time to complete than a full threshold central field, particularly in view of the relatively recent advances in threshold strategies using SITA.

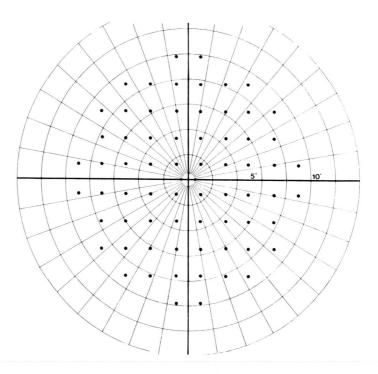

Figure 3.4 10-2 strategy. Each division on the horizontal and vertical meridia of the visual field printout represents 2 degrees. Reproduced with permission (Haley 1987).

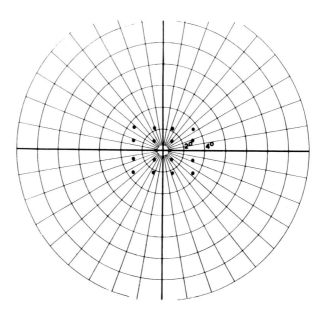

Figure 3.5 Macula strategy. Each division on the horizontal and vertical meridia of the visual field printout represents 2 degrees. Reproduced with permission (Haley 1987).

Advantages/disadvantages

In screening programmes, a larger number of points may be tested in a shorter period of time unless the field is abnormal; this is less demanding for the patient. In threshold programmes more information is obtained relating to the defects and their depth; this is more time consuming. With new programmes including the SITA software, tests have speeded up considerably, so a SITA fast strategy will give a threshold test result in a shorter period of time than some central screening programmes. SITA standard and fast are designed to run with the following threshold programmes: central 30-2, 24-2, 10-2 and peripheral 60-4 on the series 7 analyser. All tests must use a white size III stimulus.

24-2 versus 30-2 programme

The 24-2 and 30-2 programmes are commonly employed in clinical practice. However, there has been debate as to which should be used preferentially (Anderson 1992; Fingeret 1995; Khoury *et al.* 1999). In threshold static perimetry, the number of locations tested determines test time. The amount of diagnostic information increases with the number of locations tested, although the extra information from each additional test point diminishes as the number of test points increases. Perimetry of the area outside the central 30 degrees is often unreliable, time consuming, difficult for the patient and has high test–retest variability. The 24-2 or 30-2 programmes are therefore most preferable.

The 24-2 full threshold programme tests the central 24 degrees of the visual field but includes the nasal field to 30 degrees, and tests 54 points with a 6 degree spaced grid offset from the vertical and horizontal meridians. The 30-2 full threshold programme tests the central 30 degrees of the visual field and tests 76 points with a 6 degree spaced grid offset from the vertical and horizontal meridians. However, the main disadvantage is that the 30-2 requires a longer testing time. One way to reduce test time is to decrease the number of test points. A larger increment between successive test stimuli also may improve the reproducibility of the threshold determination by reducing physiological fatigue (American Academy of Ophthalmology 1996).

With regard to the test pattern, some advocate that the test be shortened by testing a grid of only 54 points that cover only the central 24 degrees of the visual field plus two extra points located 27 degrees nasally. The argument is that abnormalities and changes confined to the edge ring of points in the central 30-2 pattern are often ignored as non-specific so there is little reason to test these locations. The counter argument is that with the 24-2 pattern, at the conclusion of the examination there is a new rim of edge points that may have isolated and therefore uncertain abnormalities (Anderson 1992).

Colour perimetry

This form of visual field assessment can be used for testing macular sensitivity, with red or green targets. Assessment of the normal red field is between

5 and 7 degrees and the green field between 3 and 5 degrees from the central point of fixation. Conditions in which these fields may be performed include: patients taking hydroxychloroquine for arthritic conditions, compressive thyroid eye disease and optic neuritis (Easterbrook & Trope 1989; Hart *et al.* 1995). Common programmes used in colour perimetry are the 10 degree and macular 4 degree programmes.

Coloured targets may be presented on a white background or on a coloured background. The latter eliminates two of the three colour systems by selective adaptation using the appropriate background colour. This therefore allows determination of perimetric threshold for one single colour system.

Glaucoma is thought to selectively affect the blue cone mechanism and can produce more significant defects when blue stimuli are used on a yellow background (Simunovic *et al.* 2004). Humphrey perimetry allows blue-on-yellow perimetry (short wavelength automated perimetry; SWAP). A yellow background desensitises

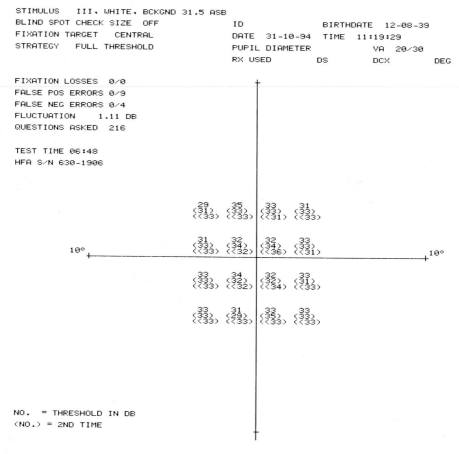

Figure 3.6 Macula threshold visual field assessment; hydroxychloroquine therapy. The visual field result shows both right and left eyes with threshold sensitivity in decibel values and defect depth in decibel values. The left eye has a normal result. The right eye shows some loss in sensitivity at three points.

red and green cones, thereby allowing assessment of blue cones which are most susceptible to change in glaucoma. Blue–yellow defects precede those in white-on-white perimetry and are larger (Sample & Weinreb 1990, 1992; Johnson *et al.* 1992/1993, 1993). This form of assessment is not used routinely as results can be affected by lens opacities and it is more difficult for the patient than conventional perimetry, thereby increasing variability.

Macular and central threshold programmes

The macular programme may also be used to test the central area using white targets within the central 4 degrees and the 10-2 programme used for the central 10 degrees. This assessment should be undertaken for specific reported central defects or if the peripheral field is so constricted that only a small central area of vision remains. Figure 3.6 shows the results of a macular threshold test in a patient taking hydroxychloroquine.

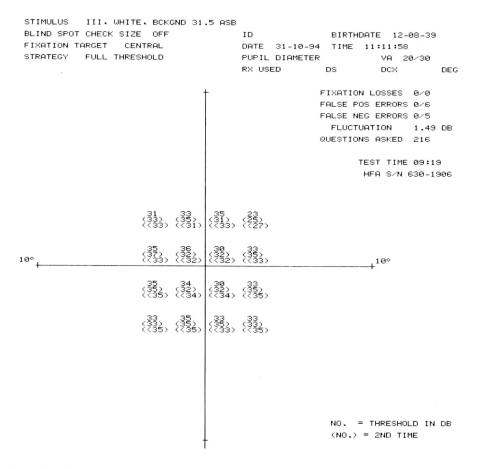

Figure 3.6 (Continued)

Esterman strategy

The Esterman programme should be used for Driver and Vehicle Licensing Agency (DVLA) driving visual field assessments, and may be performed as a binocular or monocular test dependent on the patient's visual acuity in either eye.

The target size is equivalent to a size III Goldmann target and the target intensity is 10 decibels. The binocular programme assesses 120 points and extends 75 degrees nasally, 75 degrees temporally, 40 degrees superiorly and 60 degrees inferiorly (Fig. 3.7). The monocular programme assesses 100 points and extends 60 degrees nasally, 75 degrees temporally, 40 degrees superiorly and 60 degrees inferiorly (Fig. 3.8). More points are concentrated within the central 40 degrees of the visual field than in the peripheral field.

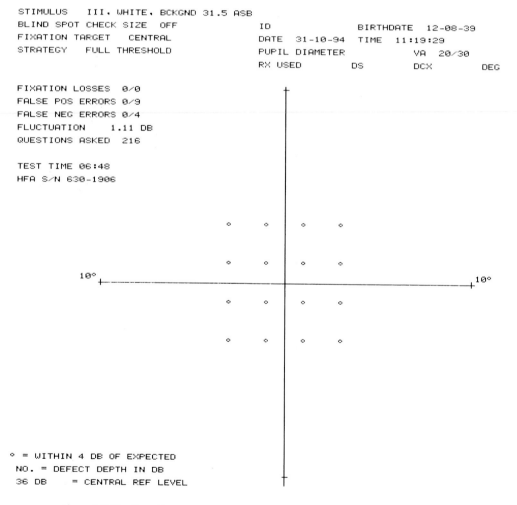

Figure 3.6 (Continued)

When testing the binocular Esterman, assessment of reliability does not include assessment of fixation losses as the blind spots cannot be checked. However, fixation may be monitored visually by the examiner, and the perimeter will continue to assess false positive and false negative responses by presenting stimuli in previously assessed areas. False negative responses may relate to areas of visual loss as there is no response to a stimulus in an area which has generated a prior response. False positive responses occur when the patient makes a response in the absence of stimulus. Visual fields demonstrating more than 20% of false responses should be retested as such visual fields cannot be accepted as reliable. During the process of testing the Esterman field, each point of the programme is tested twice and is only marked as an unseen point where the patient fails to respond to the stimuli on both occasions (Rowe 1998).

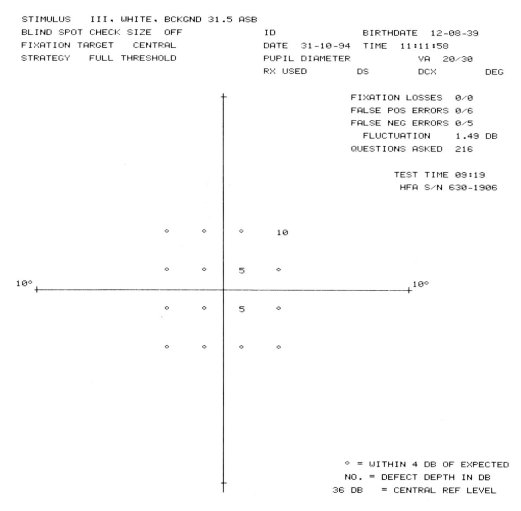

Figure 3.6 (Continued)

Fixation Monitor: OFF
Fixation Target: Central
Fixation Losses: 0/0
False POS Errors: 0/10
False NEG Errors: 0/8
Test Duration: 03:56

Stimulus Intensity: 10 dB

Stimulus: III, White
Background: 31.5 ASB
Strategy: Two Zone
Test Mode: Single Intensity

Pupil Diameter:
Visual Acuity:
RX: DS   DC X

Date: 07-10-99
Time: 12:10
Age: 20

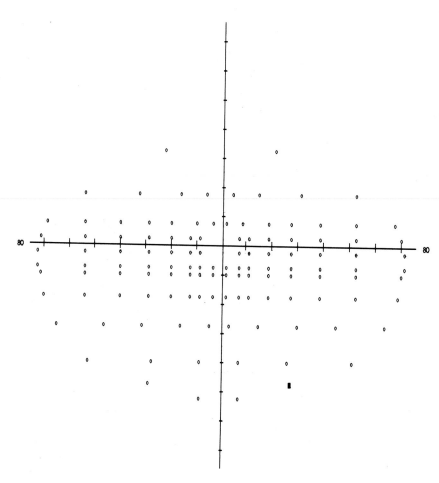

o Seen 119/120
∎ Not Seen 1/120
△ Blindspot
Esterman Efficiency Score: 99

Figure 3.7 Binocular Esterman programme. The acceptable binocular result is 120 degrees along the horizontal meridian and 20 degrees above and below the horizontal meridian with no defect within the central 40 degrees.

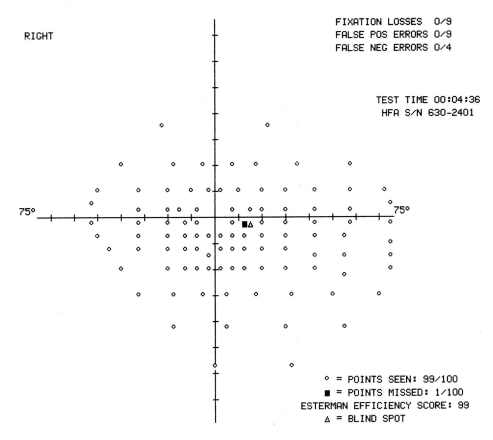

Figure 3.8 Monocular Esterman programme. The acceptable monocular result is 100 degrees along the horizontal meridian and 20 degrees above and below the horizontal meridian with no defect within the central 40 degrees.

Visual standards for safe driving

The level of visual acuity required for driving is equivalent to 6/10 (Rowe 1998). UK law states that 'A licence holder or applicant is suffering a prescribed disability if unable to meet the eyesight requirements, i.e. to read in good light (with the aid of glasses or contact lenses if worn) a registration mark fixed to a motor vehicle and containing letters and figures 79 millimetres high and 57 millimetres wide at a distance of 20.5 metres or 79 millimetres high and 50 millimetres wide at a distance of 20 metres. If unable to meet this standard the driver must not drive and the licence must be refused or revoked.'

A good field of vision is also required, and accurate and reliable assessment of the visual field is important in order to ascertain whether the degree of visual field meets the requirements for driving. The DVLA states that an adequate field of vision is required by law and a considerable deterioration in the binocular field of vision is a hazardous defect (Johnson & Keltner 1983). Drivers with restricted fields may be prone to a higher incidence of side collisions.

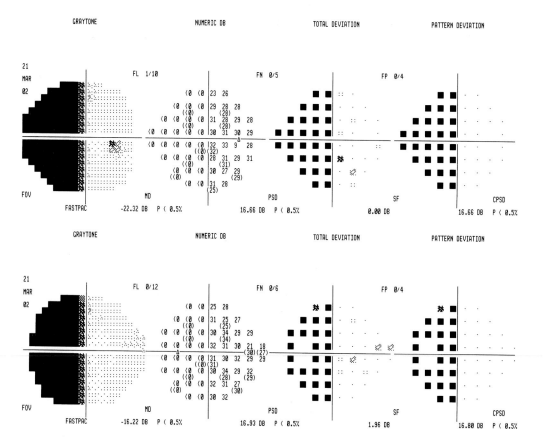

Figure 3.9 Esterman visual field assessment; hemianopia. There is a left homonymous hemianopia which is evident on the 24-2 central threshold visual field result for both right and left eyes in addition to the binocular Esterman result.

The minimum field of vision for safe driving is defined as 'a field of at least 120 degrees on the horizontal measured using a target equivalent to the white Goldmann III4e settings. In addition, there should be no significant defect in the binocular field which encroaches within 20 degrees of fixation above or below the horizontal meridian. Homonymous or bitemporal defects which come close to fixation, whether hemianopic or quadrantanopic, are not accepted as safe for driving.'

The DVLA requires a binocular Esterman field to determine fitness to drive. Monocular full field charts may also be requested in specific conditions. Monocular vision is not a cause for disqualification as long as the visual field is normal in the remaining eye. The exception to this is that monocular drivers are permitted to drive even though their physiological blind spot constitutes a field defect within the central 20 degrees of fixation.

In both binocular and monocular Esterman results, the false positive score must be no more than 20%. Fixation accuracy must be considered.

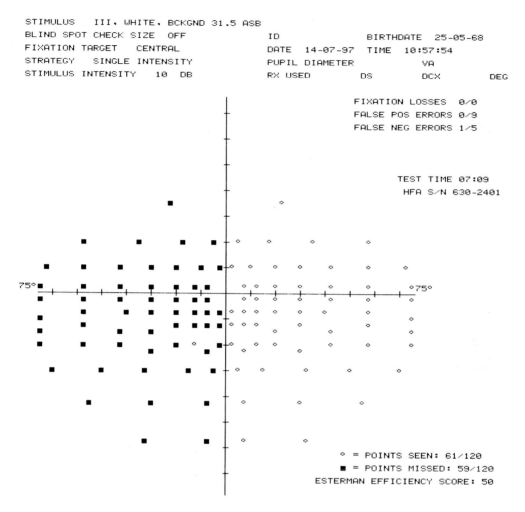

```
STIMULUS    III, WHITE, BCKGND 31.5 ASB
BLIND SPOT CHECK SIZE   OFF          ID              BIRTHDATE   25-05-68
FIXATION TARGET    CENTRAL           DATE  14-07-97  TIME   10:57:54
STRATEGY    SINGLE INTENSITY         PUPIL DIAMETER           VA
STIMULUS INTENSITY    10  DB         RX USED        DS      DCX        DEG
```

FIXATION LOSSES   0/0
FALSE POS ERRORS 0/9
FALSE NEG ERRORS 1/5

TEST TIME 07:09
HFA S/N 630-2401

75° — 75°

○ = POINTS SEEN: 61/120
■ = POINTS MISSED: 59/120
ESTERMAN EFFICIENCY SCORE: 50

Figure 3.9 (Continued)

Acceptable central loss for Group 1 drivers includes scattered single missed points and a single cluster of up to three contiguous points. Unacceptable central loss includes a cluster of four or more contiguous points that is either wholly or partly within the central 20 degree area, loss consisting of both a single cluster of three contiguous missed points up to and including 20 degrees from fixation and any additional separate missed point(s) within the central 20 degree area, and central loss of any size that is an extension of a hemianopia or quadrantanopia.

It is the practitioner's responsibility to advise patients suspected of having a notifiable eye condition or a visual field defect to declare this to the DVLA. The DVLA then issues a questionnaire to the patient and on completion, the DVLA requests further details of the eye condition from the ophthalmologist who completes a form stating whether or not visual standards for driving are met. Drivers with visual field defects who fail to notify the DVLA are committing a criminal offence.

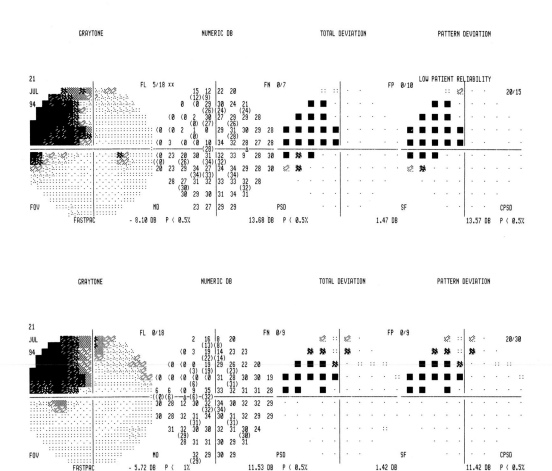

Figure 3.10 Esterman visual field assessment; quadrantanopia. There is a left superior homonymous quadrantanopia which is evident on the 30-2 central threshold visual field result for both right and left eyes in addition to the binocular Esterman result.

Interpretation

Monocular Esterman driving tests will usually reflect the monocular central threshold test results. However, binocular Esterman driving tests may or may not reflect the monocular threshold results. In general, homonymous hemianopic or quadrantanopic visual field defects will be recorded by both monocular threshold and binocular Esterman tests (Figs 3.9 and 3.10). These commonly relate to post chiasmal lesions of the visual pathway.

Lesions of the optic nerve and optic chiasm resulting in marked visual field defects on monocular threshold tests may not appear as marked on binocular testing of the visual field, and on occasion may provide a driving test result which apparently meets the standards of the DVLA. One example of this is a patient with glaucoma who has visual field loss involving the superior field of one eye and the inferior field of the other eye. The visual loss in glaucoma predominantly involves the nasal

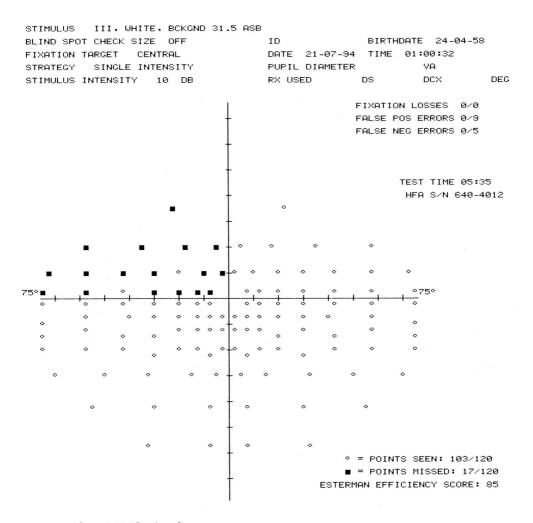

Figure 3.10 (Continued)

field; in such cases either eye may compensate for each other and provide a normal or near normal result on binocular assessment which conforms to the DVLA standards. These results are often acceptable, but the visual status of the patient must be monitored to detect any further progression of the condition with subsequent change in the visual field (Rowe 1998).

An apparently normal driving field may also be obtained in optic chiasm disease. Bitemporal hemianopias of varying degree are documented with optic chiasm disease due to pituitary tumours, craniopharyngioma, vascular lesions or any other lesion of the optic chiasm and sellar region. Monocular visual field tests will demonstrate temporal defects clearly. However, on binocular tests, the nasal visual fields of either eye may compensate for the lack of temporal field response, and a near normal response can be obtained which appears to conform to DVLA driving standards. Such a case is not, however, acceptable for driving standards; where information on visual fields of such a case is required, both monocular test results and the binocular driving test should be provided (Rowe 1998).

The Esterman test may also fail drivers unfairly. Those patients with visual field loss in one eye and normal visual field in the other may, in some cases, not provide an acceptable binocular Esterman result. The test may show a missed point in the area of the blind spot of the normal eye, where the other eye has not compensated for this. Where such a query exists, it is advisable to repeat the Esterman monocularly for the normal eye, as a normal monocular field of vision meets the DVLA driving standards.

Patients with other conditions such as those relating to retinopathy (e.g. segmental retinitis pigmentosa) may have a borderline result on Esterman testing,

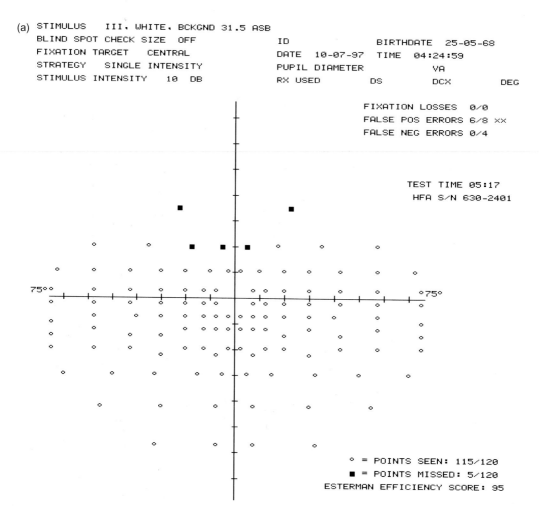

Figure 3.11 Esterman and Goldmann perimeter visual field assessments: sector retinitis pigmentosa. The binocular Esterman result (a) shows encroachment of the central 20 degree visual field; Goldmann result (b) shows superior sector visual field loss along this margin.

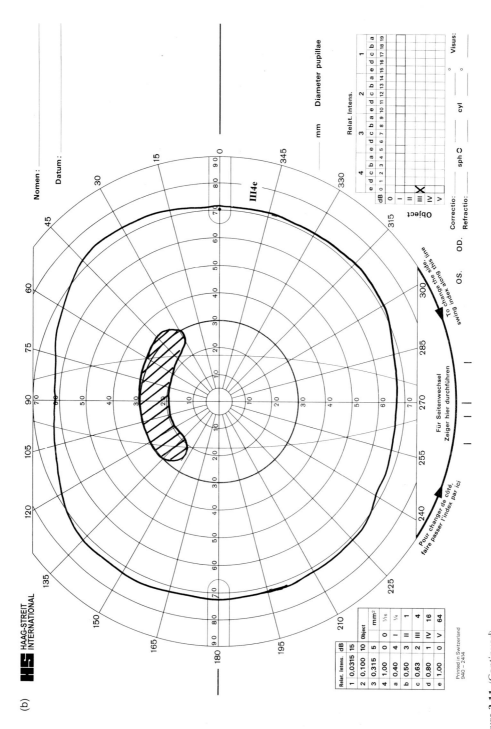

Figure 3.11 (Continued)

where the visual field loss encroaches on the area of visual field required by DVLA standards. Further assessment of the visual field with a perimeter such as the Goldmann manual perimeter may provide more information on the central and peripheral visual field (Fig. 3.11). The ophthalmologist may then forward this information to the DVLA for individual consideration.

Choice of visual field assessment

A monocular Esterman test is suitable for monocular drivers. A binocular Esterman test is recommended for all binocularly sighted drivers. Bilateral monocular Esterman tests may also be required, but there are no specific criteria as to when a monocular test is advisable in addition to the binocular test. Bilateral monocular tests should be considered where there is severe bilateral disease, such as bitemporal hemianopia, in order to document fully the extent of the monocular fields in comparison to the binocular field. Bilateral monocular fields are also recommended where there is reduced visual acuity of less than 6/60 in one eye but with a full field; where there is reduced visual acuity of less than 6/24 with moderate contraction of the field, aphakia or media opacities; and where there is visual acuity of 6/18 or better but with severe marked field loss. In these cases, a normal monocular field of the better eye may be obtained where the binocular result is abnormal (Rowe 1998).

References

American Academy of Ophthalmology (1996) Automated perimetry. *Ophthalmology*, **103**: 1144

Anderson DR (1992) *Automated Static Perimetry*. St Louis, CV Mosby

Easterbrook M, Trope G (1989) Value of Humphrey perimetry in the detection of early chloroquine retinopathy. *Lens and Eye Toxic Research*, **6**: 255

Fingeret M (1995) Clinical alternative for reducing the time needed to perform automated threshold perimetry. *Journal of American Optometry Association*, **66**: 699

Haley MJ (1987) *The Field Analyzer Primer*, 2nd edn. CA, Allergan, Humphrey

Hart WM, Kosmorsky G, Burde RM (1995) Color perimetry of central scotomas in diseases of the macula and optic nerve. *Documenta Ophthalmogica Proceedings Series*, **42**: 239

Heijl A, Patella VM (2002) *The Field Analyzer Primer. Essential Perimetry*, 3rd edn. Dublin, CA, Carl Zeiss Meditec

Johnson CA, Adams AJ, Casson EJ (1992/1993) Blue-on-yellow perimetry; a five-year overview. In: *Perimetry Update* (ed. Mills RP). Amsterdam, Kugler & Ghedini; p. 459

Johnson CA, Adams AJ, Casson EJ, Brandt JD (1993) Blue-on-yellow perimetry can predict the development of glaucomatous visual field loss. *Archives of Ophthalmology*, **111**: 645

Johnson CA, Keltner JL (1983) Incidence of visual field loss in 20,000 eyes and its relationship to driving performance. *Archives of Ophthalmology*, **101**: 371

Khoury JM, Donahue SP, Lavin PJ, Tsai JC (1999) Comparison of 24-2 and 30-2 perimetry in glaucomatous and nonglaucomatous optic neuropathies. *Journal of NeuroOphthalmology*, **19**: 100

Rowe FJ (1998) Esterman driving tests using Humphrey automated perimetry. *British Orthoptic Journal*, **55**: 57

Sample PA, Weinreb RN (1990) Color perimetry for assessment of primary open angle glaucoma. *Investigative Ophthalmology and Visual Science* **31**: 1869

Sample PA, Weinreb RN (1992) Progressive color visual field loss in glaucoma. *Investigative Ophthalmology and Visual Science,* **33**: 2068

Simunovic MP, Cullerne A, Colley A, Wilson TD (2004) How well does color perimetry isolate responses from individual cone mechanisms? *Journal of Glaucoma,* **13**: 22

Further reading

Asman P, Heijl A (1992) Evaluation of methods for automated hemifield analysis in perimetry. *Archives of Ophthalmology,* 110: 820

Hobbs HE, Sorsby A, Freedman A (1959) Retinopathy following chloroquine therapy. *Lancet,* **2**: 478

Keltner JL, Johnson CA. (1980) Mass visual field screening in a driving population. *Ophthalmology,* **89**: 785

Mindel JS, Safir A, Schara PW (1983) Visual field testing with red targets. *Archives of Ophthalmology,* **101**: 927

Rowe FJ (1998) Visual field analysis with Humphrey automated perimetry. Parts I and II. *Eye News,* 4(6) 6–10; 5(1) 15–19

Rowe FJ (1999) *Idiopathic intracranial hypertension. Assessment of visual function and prognosis for visual outcome,* PhD thesis, APU Cambridge

Sample PA, Taylor JD, Martinez GA, Lusky M, Weinreb RN (1993) Short-wavelength color visual fields in glaucoma suspects at risk. *American Journal of Ophthalmology,* **115**: 225

Siatkowski RM, Lam B, Anderson DR, Feuer WJ, Halikman AM (1996) Automated suprathreshold static perimetry screening in neuro-ophthalmology. *Ophthalmology,* **103**: 907

Steel SE, Mackie SW, Walsh G (1996) Visual field defects due to spectacle frames: their prediction and relationship to UK driving standards. *Ophthalmic and Physiological Optics,* **16**: 95

Taylor JF (ed.) (1995) *Medical Aspects of Fitness to Drive. A Guide for Medical Practitioners.* London, Medical Commission on Accident Prevention

Weiner A, Sandberg MA, Gaudio AR, Kini MM, Berson EL (1991) Hydroxychloroquine retinopathy. *American Journal of Ophthalmology,* **112**: 528

Chapter 4

Ocular media

The ocular media comprise all 'clear' structures of the eye through which light rays pass to reach the retina, i.e. cornea, aqueous fluid, anterior chamber, lens, vitreous fluid and posterior chamber.

CORNEA

Anatomy*

The cornea is the transparent area at the front of the eyeball continuous with the sclera. It is composed of five layers:

(1) Outer surface epithelium
(2) Bowman's layer
(3) Stroma
(4) Descemet's membrane
(5) Inner surface endothelium.

The epithelium is a non-keratinised stratified squamous epithelium. Bowman's layer is an acellular layer consisting of fine interwoven collagen fibrils. The stroma comprises the majority of the cornea and consist of flattened lamellae composed of collagen fibrils with flattened stellate cells between the lamellae. Descemet's membrane is a modified basement membrane of the endothelium and is composed of basement membrane glycoproteins, laminin and collagen in a lattice arrangement. The endothelium is a single layer of flattened hexagonal-shaped cells.

A healthy clear ocular surface is essential for corneal refraction and transparency. The cornea and associated tear film are the main refractive media of the eye. The cornea is transparent due to the regular arrangement of the outer epithelium, regular arrangement of the stromal collagen fibrils and avascularity. As the cornea is avascular it receives nutrients by diffusion from the aqueous humour and capillaries at its margins.

---

*The anatomy sections in this chapter are intended as a brief description only. If required, further detail should be sought from appropriate textbooks – see Further reading. The anatomy and pathology sections, in combination, provide a background to the part of the visual pathway covered in this chapter so that the relevant visual field defects can be considered and interpreted appropriately.

Pathology*

Congenital abnormalities

Congenital anomalies include abnormalities of size, abnormalities of curvature and opacities.

Acquired abnormalities

Corneal degeneration

Degeneration of the cornea may be caused, for example, by pterygium which are fleshy vascular growths extending from the conjunctiva onto the cornea and are caused by light damage.

Corneal dystrophies

These may be anterior (epithelial), stromal, posterior or ectatic (keratoconus).

Anterior dystrophies can be due to recurrent erosions. Stromal dystrophies involve accumulation of deposits in the stromal layer, e.g. granular dystrophy, macular dystrophy, lattice dystrophy. Posterior dystrophies involve Decesmet's membrane and the endothelium, e.g. corneal guttata. Corneal dystrophy may be secondary to systemic disease, e.g. Fuch's dystrophy.

Corneal oedema

There is accumulation of fluid in the stroma and epithelium due to a failure of endothelium function which can be caused by a dystrophy, trauma, glaucoma or following surgical grafting procedures.

Inflammation/infection

Infections of the outer eye can result in corneal opacities and haze (e.g. viral, herpes simplex (Colour Plate 4.1), trachoma, bacterial, parasitic disease and infestations). Corneal scarring can be caused by trichiasis (lashes are turned inwards against the eye). Ulcers such as herpes simplex ulcer, if not treated appropriately, can lead to permanent visual loss. Contact lens related keratitis can lead to corneal abscess. Allergic reactions can also result in corneal haze and ulcers.

Inflammation of the cornea (keratitis) may be infectious (viruses, chlamydia, bacteria) or non-infectious (trauma, burns).

---

*The pathology sections in this chapter are provided as a summary of possible disease processes but by their nature cannot be all inclusive. The reader is directed towards other appropriate textbooks for further detail – see Further reading.

Orbital mass

A mass around or behind the eye resulting in proptosis of the eye can result in corneal damage due to exposure of the cornea with inadequate lid coverage.

Trauma

Trauma may directly involve the cornea with a penetrating injury or a chemical eye injury.

Associated signs and symptoms*

Patients may have a clear history of trauma or medical problems. Anterior segment examination will show features of corneal involvement dependent on the pathology present. Use of staining agents will highlight pathology, such as corneal ulcers.

Patients will be aware of a loss or reduction in their vision. Patients with corneal infections and/or inflammation often present with a painful, photophobic red eye. Those patients with thyroid eye disease complain of pain, grittyness, diplopia and blurred vision. General symptoms are also present. Ocular signs include chemosis, lid retraction and strabismus. Thyroid eye disease patients can have visual loss due to corneal exposure, but more important is the visual loss that occurs from orbital apex compression of the optic nerve by the enlarged extraocular muscles.

ANTERIOR CHAMBER

Anatomy

The anterior chamber is an area between the posterior surface of the cornea and anterior surface of the lens, and is filled with clear fluid (aqueous humour). Aqueous fluid is produced by the ciliary body, passes forward in the anterior chamber and predominantly is drained through the trabecular meshwork in the angle of the cornea and sclera (limbal area).

Secretion of aqueous humour generates the intraocular pressure required for an optically efficient globe, and pressure is normally maintained between 10 and 20 mmHg (but varies according to age).

Pathology

The clarity of the aqueous humour can be altered by deposits within the fluid. Inflammation/infectious processes result in cell deposits within the aqueous humour that cloud the fluid (Colour Plate 4.2). Haemorrhage following trauma such as with hyphaema will cloud the aqueous fluid.

---

*The sections on associated signs and symptoms are provided so that the practitioner is aware of additional information that can be considered in conjunction with the visual field defect to aid differential diagnosis and localisation of pathology.

Associated signs and symptoms

In acute anterior uveitis (inflammation) there is usually a dull ocular and/or peri-orbital pain, photophobia and a mild reduction in vision. Ciliary injection may be evident and the patient may have a hypopyon. Keratitic precipitates are deposits of fibrin and cells on the corneal endothelium.

Dense clouding of the aqueous fluid, as with haemorrhage, will result in a marked loss of vision. Deposits within the aqueous fluid can be graded according to the severity of clouding (flare) in the anterior chamber.

LENS

Anatomy

The lens is a transparent biconvex structure situated between the iris and vitreous humour. It is attached by zonules to the ciliary body. It consists of:

(1) Lens capsule
(2) Lens epithelium
(3) Lens fibres and sutures.

The lens capsule is a thickened basement membrane that envelops the entire lens. It is produced by the lens epithelium anteriorly and the superficial lens fibres posteriorly. It consists of collagen fibrils embedded in a matrix of glycoproteins and sulphated glycosaminoglycans. Zonular fibres that connect the lens to the ciliary processes are inserted into the region of the equator. The adult lens is approximately 10 mm in diameter and 4 mm thick. It continues to grow throughout life. The lens epithelium is a simple cuboidal epithelium restricted to the anterior surface of the lens. The lens fibres constitute the main mass of the lens and are formed by the multiplication and differentiation of the lens epithelial cells at the equator.

After the age of 40–50 years the elasticity of the lens markedly decreases. Transmission of light decreases with age and there is increased degradation of lens proteins, and increase in sodium and calcium concentrations.

Pathology

Congenital abnormalities

Congenital anomalies include aphakia, cataract and lenticonus. Congenital cataract may be due to genetic, metabolic or chromosome defects.

Acquired abnormalities

Cataract (Colour Plate 4.3)

Lens opacification is the response of the lens to any insult that disturbs normal development or metabolism. Acquired cataract may be primary or secondary and may be senile or due to endocrine, trauma, metabolic or disease processes. Cataracts take many forms including mature, nuclear sclerotic, cortical lens opacity, posterior subcapsular lens opacity and traumatic.

Ectopic lens

The lens is displaced eccentrically from its usual central position behind the iris, e.g. Marfan's syndrome.

Associated signs and symptoms

There is a generalised loss or impairment of visual function with cataract. Reduced vision is caused by increased light scatter. In the early stages this may be a reduction in contrast sensitivity and colour sensitivity, but progresses to loss of high contrast visual acuity.

Lens pathology is evident on anterior segment examination using the slit-lamp. Such examination also allows the differentiation of cataract types and the grading of the extent of cataract change.

An eccentrically displaced lens will result in marked astigmatic refractive errors which impair clarity of visual acuity. Conditions such as Marfan's syndrome have additional general signs such as increased stature and long digits.

POSTERIOR CHAMBER

Anatomy

The posterior chamber is an area behind the lens and is filled with clear fluid (vitreous humour). The vitreous humour occupies approximately two-thirds of the globe by volume. The posterior chamber is spherical but anteriorly has a saucer shaped depression for the lens (the hyaloid fossa). It is bound anteriorly by the lens and ciliary body, and posteriorly by the retina. The composition of vitreous fluid is approximately 98% water, the remainder being hyaluronate and collagen. A fine network of collagen fibres provides structure.

Pathology

Congenital abnormalities

Congenital anomalies include persistent primary vitreous and persistent hyperplastic primary vitreous.

Acquired abnormalities

Acquired anomalies include vitreous adhesions, vitreous opacities and inflammation, haemorrhage or cells within the vitreous.

Vitreous detachment can occur independently or prior to retinal detachment. There is potential space between the vitreous and the lens and between the vitreous and the retina where fluid can accumulate in pathological conditions. Degeneration with age can lead to vitreous detachment which then predisposes to retinal detachment. Detachment of the vitreous from the retina increases traction which can lead to a retina break.

Vitreous haemorrhage may result from trauma or may be spontaneous due to retinal tears, or neovascular with posterior vitreous detachment and central retinal vein occlusion.

Associated signs and symptoms

Acquired vitreous pathology is associated with sudden painless visual loss. Patients may be aware of numerous tiny floaters seen prior to the loss of vision. Pathology may be documented using slit-lamp examination or by indirect ophthalmoscopy.

VISUAL FIELD DEFECTS

It is not common practice to undertake visual field assessment in cases of visual disturbance by media opacities. There is no specific visual field defect to be plotted, but merely an interruption of the visual field perception by the various opacities commonly resulting in a general reduction in sensitivity. Many conditions are treatable and once successful treatment has been received, the patient's visual capacity returns to normal.

Any opacity of the ocular media reduces test object illumination. For example, miosis will magnify the effect of a cataract. When interpreting visual field defects in an eye with media opacities, adequate allowance must be made for the opacity's

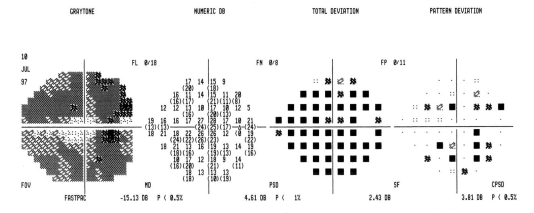

Figure 4.1 Humphrey perimeter visual field assessment: cataract. There is reduced sensitivity across the field of vision. Note the reduced decibel values and the reduction in total deviation probability plot. The corrected pattern standard deviation is much improved but with some deficit requiring observation.

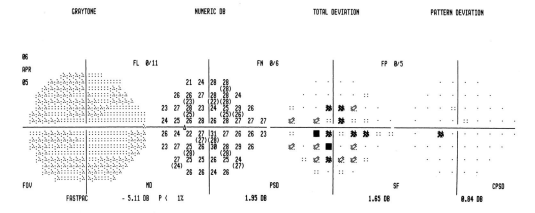

Figure 4.2 Humphrey perimeter visual field assessment: corneal dystrophy. There is reduced sensitivity of the central visual field with a reduction in total deviation plot centrally. The corrected pattern standard deviation plot is normal.

effect on the visual field result. In order to do the test, more light should be used and/or larger test objects.

One of the most common pathologies is that of cataract which causes a reduction of sensitivity across the central visual field (Fig. 4.1). With corneal dystrophy the marked corneal opacity typically causes a pronounced generalised depression of sensitivity in the central field (Fig. 4.2). In general, anterior opacities typically result in general reduction of sensitivity (due to scattered light), whereas posterior opacities result in more localised visual field defects (due to shadow effects).

It must be recognised that media opacities may occur in a patient who requires visual field assessment for another sight threatening condition. Abnormalities of media clarity are a particular problem with combined glaucoma and cataract, and when both are progressive. In such cases, it is important that all aspects of the patient's ocular status are taken into consideration, and that worsening visual fields are attributed to the correct condition which may be due to a cataract increasing in density or deteriorating glaucoma or a combination of the two.

References

Olver J, Cassidy L (2005) *Ophthalmology at a Glance*. Oxford, Blackwell Publishing.

Further reading

Adler FH, Kaufman PL (eds) (2002) *Adler's Physiology of the Eye. Clinical Application*, 10th edn. St Louis, Mosby

Guthauser V, Flammer J (1988) Quantifying visual field damage caused by cataract. *American Journal of Ophthalmology*, **106**: 480

Kanski J (2003) *Clinical Ophthalmology. A Systematic Approach*, 5th edn. London, Butterworth Heinemann

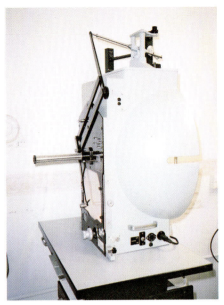

Colour Plate 2.1 Goldmann perimeter.

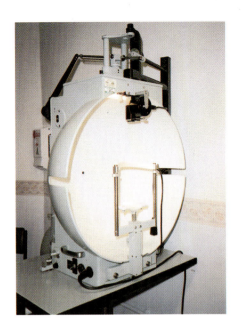

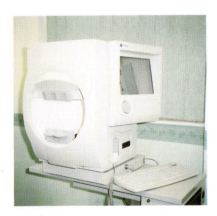

Colour Plate 2.2 Humphrey field analyser perimeter, series 7.

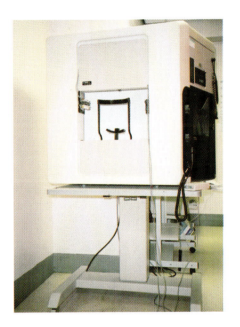

Colour Plate 3.1 Humphrey field analyser perimeter, series 6.

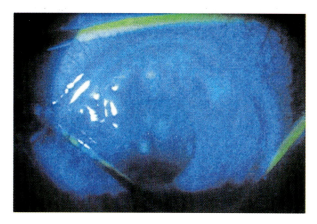

Colour Plate 4.1 Anterior segment appearance: herpes simplex virus. Note the corneal staining of the ulcer. Photograph by A. Kwan (Olver & Cassidy 2005), with permission.

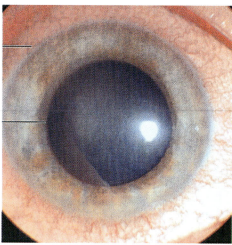

Colour Plate 4.2 Anterior segment appearance: anterior uveitis. There is some clouding of the aqueous fluid due to cell deposits with circumciliary injection. Photograph by A. Kwan (Olver & Cassidy 2005), with permission.

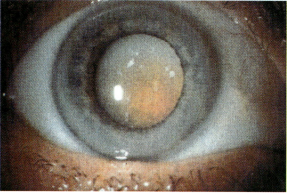

Colour Plate 4.3 Anterior segment appearance: cataract. There is dense white clouding of the lens. Photograph by A. Kwan (Olver & Cassidy 2005), with permission.

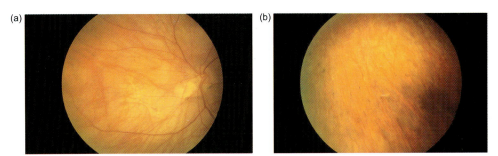

Colour Plate 5.1 Fundus appearance of retinitis pigmentosa: (a) central; (b) peripheral. The right central field is relatively spared but there is involvement of the peripheral retina.

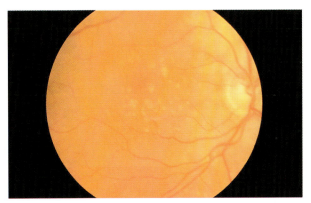

Colour Plate 5.2 Fundus appearance of macular drusen. Note the speckled appearance in the central macular area.

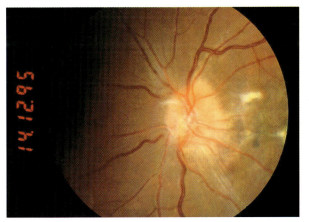

Colour Plate 5.3 Fundus appearance of toxoplasmosis. There are central changes evident on the fundus.

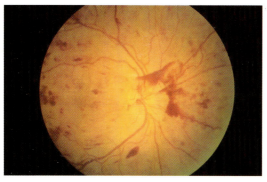

Colour Plate 5.4 Fundus appearance in diabetic retinopathy. There are multiple fundus and optic disc haemorrhages.

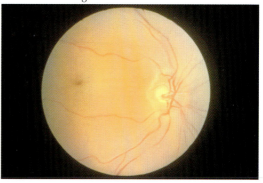

Colour Plate 5.5 Fundus appearance of central retinal artery occlusion. Note the cherry red spot at the fovea which derives its blood supply from the choroids. The avascular retina is pale in appearance.

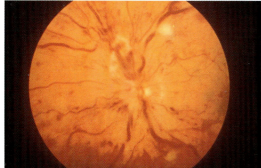

Colour Plate 5.6 Fundus appearance of central retinal vein occlusion. Note the multiple haemorrhages and tortuosity of the retinal veins.

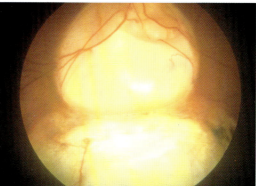

Colour Plate 6.1 Fundus appearance of coloboma. There is an enlarged excavation inferiorly with normal disc tissue located superiorly.

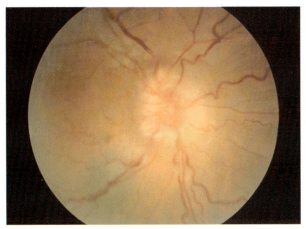

Colour Plate 6.2 Fundus appearance of optic nerve drusen. Note the enlarged swollen appearance of the disc.

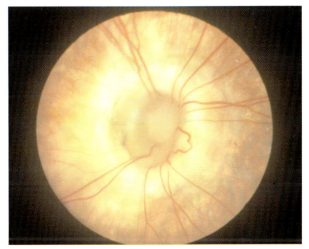

Colour Plate 6.3 Fundus appearance of morning glory syndrome. There is an enlarged and swollen appearance of the optic disc with blood vessels that emerge sharply from the rim.

(a) (b)

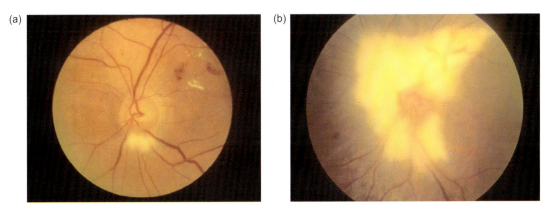

Colour Plate 6.4 Fundus appearance of myelinated nerve fibres. Myelinated nerve fibres can vary in appearance from quite minimal involvement of the nerve fibres at the optic disc (a) to quite severe involvement (b).

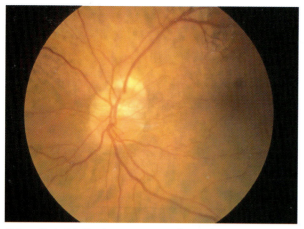

Colour Plate 6.5 Fundus appearance of optic disc pit. There is a 'double' appearance to the optic disc.

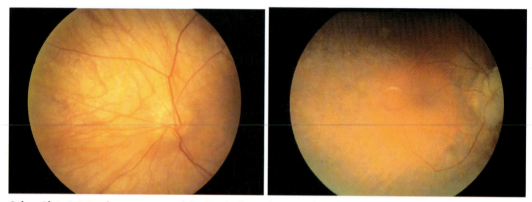

Colour Plate 6.6 Fundus appearance of tilted optic discs. There is a dragged appearance of blood vessels on the fundus.

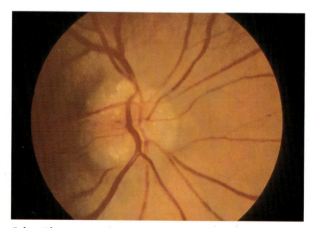

Colour Plate 6.7 Fundus appearance in optic nerve meningioma. Optic disc swelling is evident. This is the same patient as Fig. 6.2.

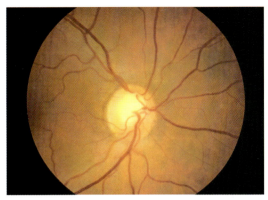

Colour Plate 6.8 Fundus appearance in glaucoma. Note the increased cup : disc ratio.

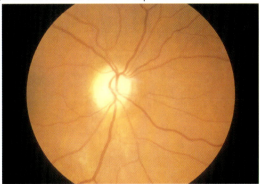

Colour Plate 6.9 Fundus appearance in optic neuritis. Severe optic neuritis can lead to optic atrophy, as evidenced by a very pale disc appearance resulting in irreversible blinding visual loss of the involved eye. Note the very pale appearance of the optic disc following an episode of optic neuritis.

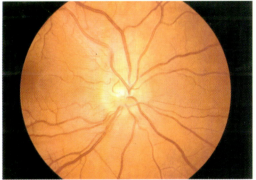

Colour Plate 6.10 Fundus appearance in early papilloedema. There is an indistinct border to the optic disc, indicating early swelling.

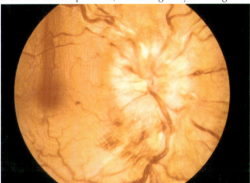

Colour Plate 6.11 Fundus appearance in acute papilloedema. Swelling has obliterated the border of the optic disc. Blood vessels are tortuous and there are numerous flame-shaped haemorrhages.

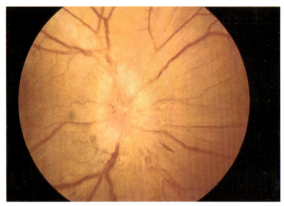

Colour Plate 6.12 Fundus appearance in chronic papilloedema. The blood vessels remain slightly tortuous. There is an indistinct border to the optic disc with advanced swelling.

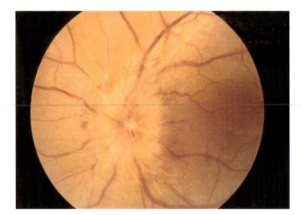

Colour Plate 6.13 Fundus appearance in vintage papilloedema. There is a bulbous appearance to the optic disc due to swelling and as a result the contents of the optic disc cannot be visualised clearly.

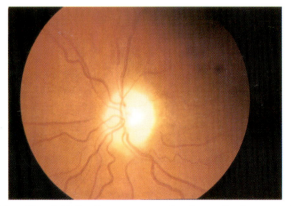

Colour Plate 6.14 Fundus appearance of optic atrophy. An extremely pale appearance of the optic disc indicates death of retinal nerve fibres.

Kanski J (2003) *Clinical Ophthalmology. A Synopsis.* London, Butterworth Heinemann/Elsevier Science

Snell RS, Lemp MA (1998) *Clinical Anatomy of the Eye*, 2nd edn. Oxford, Blackwell Publishing

Spaeth GL (1980) The management of cataract in patients with glaucoma: a comparative study I. *Transactions of the Ophthalmic Society of the UK*, **100**: 195

Chapter 5
Retina

The retina is the 'seeing' inner layer of the eye and consists of ten layers.

  (1) Pigment epithelium
  (2) Photoreceptor layer (rods and cones)
  (3) Outer limiting membrane
  (4) Outer nuclear layer
  (5) Outer plexiform layer
  (6) Inner nuclear layer
  (7) Inner plexiform layer
  (8) Layer of ganglion cells
  (9) Layer of nerve fibre axons
(10) Inner limiting membrane.

The structure differs at the fovea which consists only of the retinal pigment epithelium, photoreceptors (cones only), external limiting membrane, outer nuclear layer, inner fibres of the photoreceptors and the inner limiting membrane.

The fovea and macula pertain to the highest visual function and are located at the posterior pole of the eye. The photoreceptors synapse with bipolar cells which transmit to ganglion cells. These retinal axons converge on the optic disc (optic nerve head). The optic disc is an oval structure approximately 1.5 mm in diameter.

Each area of the retina projects to a discrete and predictable point in the striate visual cortex (V1).

There are a number of features of retinal nerve fibre arrangement that are crucial to the understanding of the production of certain visual acuity and field defects:

(1) Division between the crossed and uncrossed retinal fibres
(2) Anatomy of the temporal raphe

---

*This anatomy section is intended as a brief description only. If required, further detail should be sought from appropriate textbooks – see Further reading. The anatomy and pathology sections, in combination, provide a background to the part of the visual pathway covered in this chapter so that the relevant visual field defects can be considered and interpreted appropriately.

(3) Location of nerve fibres within the nerve fibre layer with respect to their location of origin in the retina.

Fibres originating from ganglion cells in the retina nasal to a line drawn vertically through the fovea are predominantly crossed, while those originating from ganglion cells temporal to this line are predominantly uncrossed.

Foveal/macular fibres constitute the majority of all axons leaving the eye and form the distinct papillomacular bundle (Ballantyne 1946, Radius & Anderson 1979). The papillomacular bundle occupies almost the entire temporal side of the optic disc. Fibres from the nasal portion of the fovea proceed directly to the optic disc. Fibres from the superior and inferior portions of the fovea also project almost directly to the temporal portion of the disc, arching only slightly upward or downward around the nasal foveal fibres. Fibres from the temporal portion of the fovea initially take a vertical course superiorly and inferiorly to curve around the remainder of the foveal fibres before entering the optic disc (Fig. 5.1).

Because the central portion of the human retina develops much earlier than the periphery, the axons of peripheral temporal ganglion cells do not find a direct pathway to the optic nerve entrance. Instead they must take an arched course above and below the central portion of the retina. As a result, the temporal raphe of the human retina marks a watershed between axons of the temporal half of the macular area and axons of more peripherally situated ganglion cells (Vrabec 1966). Nerve fibres from the peripheral nasal retina pass directly to the nasal aspect of the optic disc.

(a)

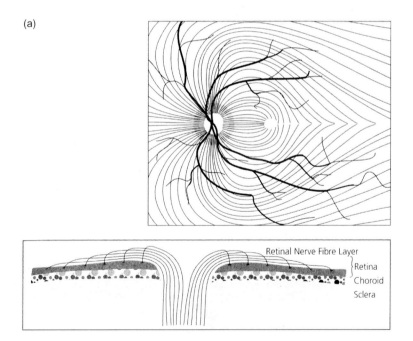

Figure 5.1 Retinal and optic disc topography. (a) Retinal ganglion fibres converge on the optic disc and are systematically layered such that longer axons from the peripheral retina are situated deeper in the retina and more peripherally in the optic disc. (b) The Goldmann chart shows the right field of vision and corresponding retinal nerve fibre distribution. Reproduced with permission (Heijl & Patella 2002).

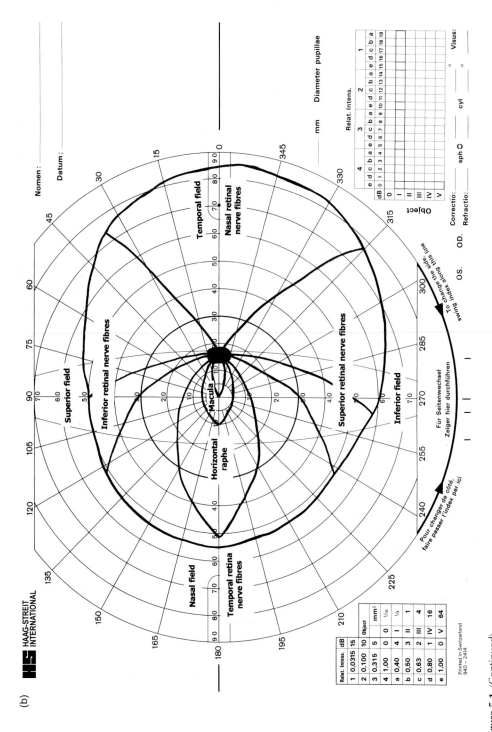

Figure 5.1 (Continued)

The retina is divided by the outer plexiform layer, so that the inner half receives its blood supply from the central retinal artery and the outer half closest to the choroid is supplied by the choroid capillaries derived from the ciliary vasculature. The central retinal artery is a branch of the ophthalmic artery and enters the eyeball with the optic nerve where it divides into two equal superior and inferior branches which in turn divide into superior and inferior nasal and temporal branches. The resulting four branches each supply a quadrant of the retina. There is no overlap of these blood vessels and no anastomosis between branches within each retinal quadrant. The fovea is supplied by an anastomosis of the central retinal artery and the choroidal circulation. The central retinal vein is formed by the union of tributaries that correspond approximately to the branches of the central artery. It leaves the eye within the optic nerve.

Pathology*

Congenital abnormalities

Congenital anomalies include albinism, pigmentation anomalies and structural abnormalities such as coloboma. Congenital tumours include von Hippel–Lindau disease and Sturge–Weber syndrome.

Acquired abnormalities

Hereditary dystrophies

Hereditary dystrophies include Stickler's syndrome and retinitis pigmentosa. **Retinitis pigmentosa** is an inherited primary retinal degeneration (Colour Plate 5.1).

Retinal degeneration

Age-related macular degeneration

This is a common retinal degeneration occurring in the elderly population. There can be a dry or wet phase. This is the commonest cause of irreversible visual loss in the developed world. There is accumulation of lipid products in Bruch's membrane due to retinal pigment epithelium cell degeneration and loss of function. This in turn results in loss of photoreceptor function.

Drusen

These are degenerative colloid bodies located between the retinal pigment epithelium and Bruch's membrane (Colour Plate 5.2).

---

*This pathology section is provided as a summary of possible disease processes but by its nature cannot be all inclusive. The reader is directed towards other appropriate textbooks for further detail – see Further reading.

Macular holes

These can be found as full or partial thickness in high myopes and solar burns. Central serous retinopathy can present with serous retinal detachment at the macula.

Retinal detachment

The neurosensory retina is susceptible to pathological separation from the underlying retinal pigment epithelium due to the presence of a tear or hole in the retina (rhegmatogenous) or due to traction or degeneration changes (non-rhegmatogenous). There is accumulation of fluid between the retinal pigment epithelium and the neurosensory retina causing the layers to separate. The separation from the underlying retinal pigment epithelium results in outer retinal degeneration.

Retinal detachment is most commonly caused by a break in the neuroepithelium with invasion of vitreous fluid into the subretinal space. As more fluid accumulates, the area and elevation of retinal separation increase. The distribution of the subretinal fluid is strongly influenced by gravity. Tears in the superior quadrants progress to total detachment more frequently than tears in the inferior quadrants.

Retinal inflammation/infection

Posterior uveitis with involvement of the retina and its vasculature can result in visual field defects. This can be caused by acquired immune deficiency syndrome (AIDS), toxoplasmosis (pigmented circumscribed scars) (Colour Plate 5.3) and toxocara. Cytomegalovirus causes an opportunistic retinal infection in patients with AIDS (Jabs 1996).

Tumours

Tumours can include choroidal neoplasms, choroidal metastasis and melanomas with involvement of retinal fibres.

Choroidal melanoma

This is the most common primary intraocular malignancy.

Choroidal naevi

These are benign asymptomatic lesions. They are flat, pigmented choroidal lesions.

Secondary metastases

These usually occur in the region of the posterior choroid; primary tumours are usually those of the breast, lung, kidney, thyroid and testis. Choroidal folds at the posterior pole are seen secondary to thyroid eye disease, orbital tumours, posterior scleritis and ocular hypotony.

Vascular abnormalities

Diabetic retinopathy

This is the most common cause of blindness in the working population. Diabetes affects the microvascular circulation in the retina (Colour Plate 5.4). Proliferative diabetic retinopathy occurs in severe cases in which new abnormal blood vessels proliferate within the eye. There is a high risk of permanent visual loss and urgent laser treatment is required. Pan-retinal laser photocoagulation is used to ablate ischaemic retina and induce regression of abnormal new vessels. Non-proliferative diabetic retinopathy is an initial stage of diabetic retinopathy and varies in severity.

Hypertensive retinopathy

This is the retinal manifestation of raised blood pressure of any cause and can produce arteriolar constriction due to autoregulation of blood flow. There is subsequent ischaemia, vascular dilatation and leakage of plasma.

Retinal vascular occlusions

Central retinal artery occlusion (Colour Plate 5.5) is most commonly caused by thrombosis in the retrobulbar portion of the central retinal artery or blockage of the artery by an embolus.

The central retinal artery is susceptible to arteriosclerotic occlusive disease which most commonly occurs at the level of the lamina cribrosa just before the artery enters the retina.

Central retinal vein occlusion (Colour Plate 5.6) may involve occlusion of the central retinal vein or a branch retinal vein with involvement of the entire field of vision, or sector, respectively.

Associated signs and symptoms*

Retinal disease tends to produce colour loss, loss of central and peripheral visual function, and impaired contrast sensitivity.

Fundus appearance

Fine pigmentary disturbance and atrophy are seen at the macula in patients with age-related macular degeneration. Fundus examination of drusen will demonstrate small yellow-white deposits in the region of the posterior pole. The retinal lesions associated with retinal infection appear as white areas with associated haemorrhages.

---

*This section on associated signs and symptoms is provided so that the practitioner is aware of additional information that can be considered in conjunction with the visual field defect to aid differential diagnosis and localisation of pathology.

Spicules of dark 'iron filings' pigmentation in the retina, arteriolar attenuation and optic disc pallor are seen in patients with retinitis pigmentosa. Persistent choroidal folds associated with ocular tumours will result in a reduction in visual function.

In vascular abnormalities, cotton wool spots which lie in the nerve fibre layer of the retina are due to ischaemic microvascular disease. Hard exudates are formed by the deposition of lipid and lipoproteins due to abnormal vascular permeability. Retinal haemorrhages may occur on the retinal surface, in the nerve fibre layer (flame-shaped), in the deeper retina (blot), under the photoreceptors or under the retinal pigment epithelium.

Macular oedema is commonly seen with posterior segment inflammation, retinal ischaemia or retinal vascular leakage. The retina has a pale appearance in central retinal artery occlusion and the fovea is temporarily seen as a cherry red spot.

Microaneurysms typify diabetic retinopathy where leakage of plasma, haemorrhage and vascular shunting occur with subsequent neovascularisation. Vessel changes such as attenuation and arteriovenous nipping are seen with haemorrhages, cotton wool spots and lipid exudates in patients with hypertensive retinopathy.

Patients with central retinal vein occlusion present with a haemorrhagic fundus, dilation of the retinal veins, retinal oedema and variable amounts of ischaemia. Branch retinal vein occlusion is limited to the affected area.

Pupil abnormalities

A relative afferent pupillary defect is seen with central retinal artery occlusion as well as other conditions causing significant loss of vision.

Visual perception

Patients with age-related macular degeneration may appreciate metamorphopsia. They have difficulty with reading and recognising faces. With macular holes, patients are aware of micropsia.

Patients with retinal detachment often present with a short history of flashes and floaters.

Retinitis pigmentosa is associated with progressive loss of night vision and constriction of the peripheral visual field. Patients can develop associated cataract or cystoid macular oedema which can further reduce vision.

With melanoma there is an awareness of flashes and floaters in the affected eye. Secondary metastases also usually present with flashes and floaters.

Complete occlusion of the central retinal artery may be preceded by attacks of amaurosis fugax.

Visual acuity

In age-related macular degeneration, patients are aware of reduced central visual acuity. With macular holes, patients are aware of blurred vision. Patients with retinal

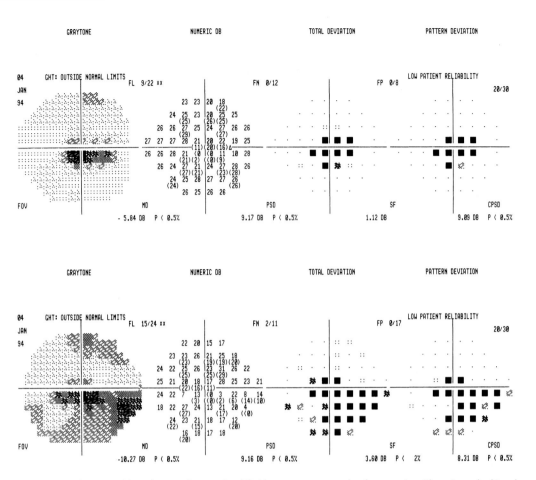

Figure 5.2 Humphrey perimeter visual field assessment: macular degeneration. There is marked involvement of the central 10 degrees of the right eye and marked involvement of the central visual field of the left eye extending to the inferior nasal visual field also.

detachment often present with a short history of reduced vision. With melanoma there is frequently reduced visual acuity. Secondary metastases usually present with visual loss in addition to advancing visual field defects.

Retinal emboli may produce permanent or temporary visual loss. In complete central artery occlusion there is a sudden onset of unilateral blindness. However, central vision can be retained if the patient has a cilioretinal artery. In branch arteriole occlusion there is partial loss of sight corresponding to the sector supplied by the arteriole. Central retinal vein occlusion can be asymptomatic if mild, but more severe cases often present with painless loss of vision of varying severity. Absorption of blood may improve visual function.

Vascular abnormalities in diabetic retinopathy may result in maculopathy with loss of visual acuity.

Visual field defects

Generally there is no pattern to the type of visual field loss seen in retinal disease processes. The variety of visual field defects produced by retinal disease is almost limitless. Visual field loss can be generalised or localised to scotomas.

Retinal degeneration

Age-related macular degeneration affects the visual field through retinal damage (Fig. 5.2). The usual visual field defect is a central scotoma of varying intensity, but often deep relative and absolute scotomas centrally. The visual field defect may be compounded by generalised depression due to cataract. Visual field defects due to drusen are dependent on the location of the lesion (Fig. 5.3).

Retinal dystrophy

Constriction of both visual fields is seen with retinal dystrophies such as retinitis pigmentosa, and occasionally from optic disc disease such as long-standing papilloedema. Deficits in retinitis pigmentosa normally start in the 20–30 degree middle zone and proceed to fixation and outward toward the periphery (Fig. 5.4). Central fixation is relatively spared. Sector retinitis pigmentosa can also occur (see Fig. 3.11) but the defects tend to cross the vertical meridian.

Retinal infection

Visual field defects are located according to the position on the retina of the pathological lesions (Fig. 5.5).

Vascular abnormalities

Altitudinal defects indicate ocular disease, and an inferior altitudinal defect is particularly a feature of anterior ischaemic optic neuropathy.

In diabetic retinopathy, visual field defects relate to non-perfused areas (scotomas). Large retinal haemorrhages may lead to relative/absolute scotomas. There is a variegated pattern of scotomas leading to a 'motheaten' appearance (Fig. 5.6).

Patients with central retinal artery occlusion typically notice monocular visual loss starting as a concentric peripheral dimming of vision or a horizontal curtain coming over the eye. Complete central retinal vein occlusion leads to generalised reduction of retinal sensitivity. Depending on the extent of haemorrhages and avascular zones there will be absolute and relative scotomas in a motheaten appearance.

Ischaemic field defects due to development of avascular areas are irreversible.

Choice of visual field assessment

The choice of perimeter or programme for visual field assessment is dependent on where the lesion is, i.e. centrally or peripherally, and also on the extent of visual acuity. Where doubt exists over the results of one programme, an alternative strategy should be considered. Where the very central area is affected, or where the very central area is all that remains, a 10-2 or macular threshold strategy should be considered.

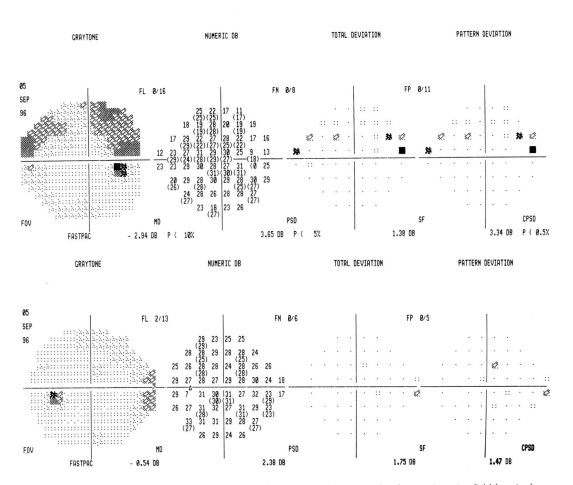

Figure 5.3 Humphrey perimeter visual field assessment: macular drusen. Superior field loss is documented in the right eye with minimal loss also documented in the macular field. The patient's visual acuities were 6/24 and 6/9.

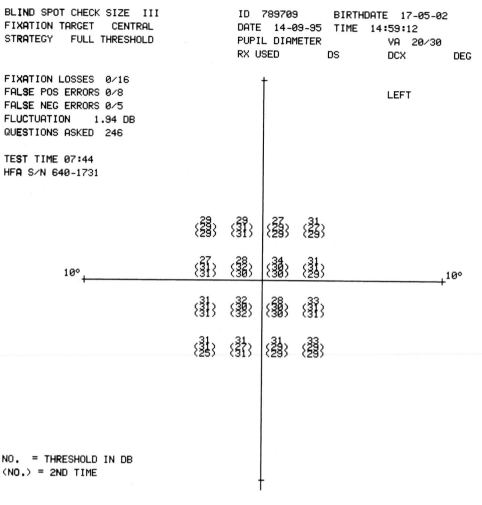

BLIND SPOT CHECK SIZE   III
FIXATION TARGET   CENTRAL
STRATEGY   FULL THRESHOLD

ID   789709   BIRTHDATE   17-05-02
DATE   14-09-95   TIME   14:59:12
PUPIL DIAMETER   VA   20/30
RX USED   DS   DCX   DEG

LEFT

FIXATION LOSSES   0/16
FALSE POS ERRORS 0/8
FALSE NEG ERRORS 0/5
FLUCTUATION   1.94 DB
QUESTIONS ASKED 246

TEST TIME 07:44
HFA S/N 640-1731

10°   10°

NO. = THRESHOLD IN DB
(NO.) = 2ND TIME

Figure 5.3 (Continued)

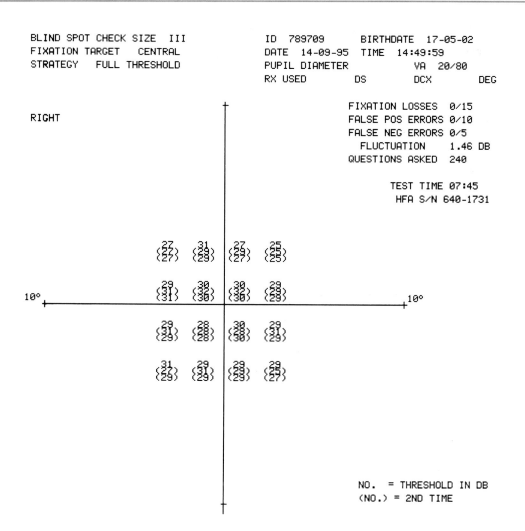

Figure 5.3 (Continued)

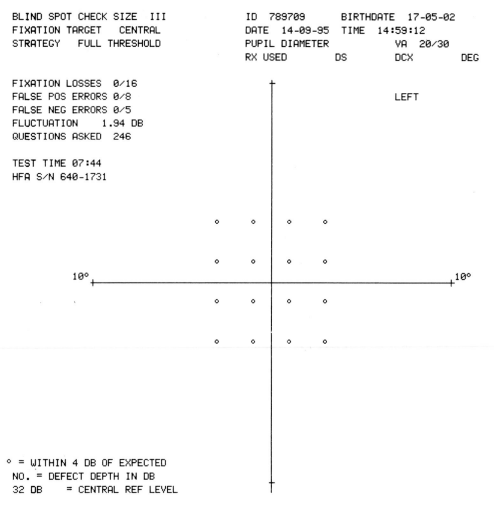

Figure 5.3 (Continued)

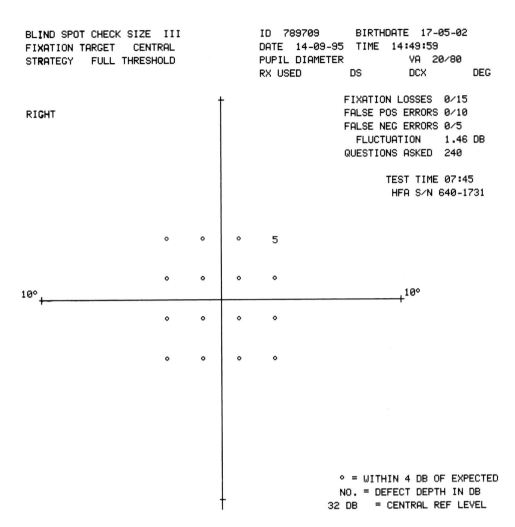

BLIND SPOT CHECK SIZE   III
FIXATION TARGET   CENTRAL
STRATEGY   FULL THRESHOLD

ID   789709   BIRTHDATE   17-05-02
DATE   14-09-95 TIME   14:49:59
PUPIL DIAMETER   VA 20/80
RX USED   DS   DCX   DEG

RIGHT

FIXATION LOSSES   0/15
FALSE POS ERRORS 0/10
FALSE NEG ERRORS 0/5
   FLUCTUATION   1.46 DB
QUESTIONS ASKED   240

TEST TIME 07:45
HFA S/N 640-1731

5

10°   10°

° = WITHIN 4 DB OF EXPECTED
NO. = DEFECT DEPTH IN DB
32 DB   = CENTRAL REF LEVEL

Figure 5.3 (Continued)

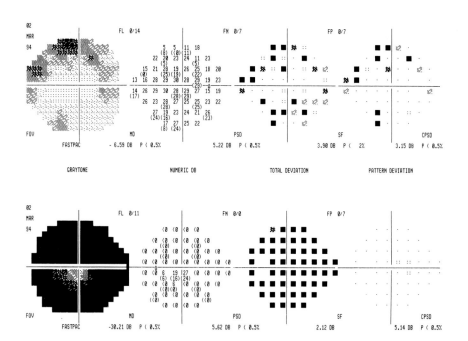

Figure 5.4 Humphrey perimeter visual field assessment: retinitis pigmentosa. There is blinding visual loss in the left eye, but a relatively spared central field remains in the right eye.

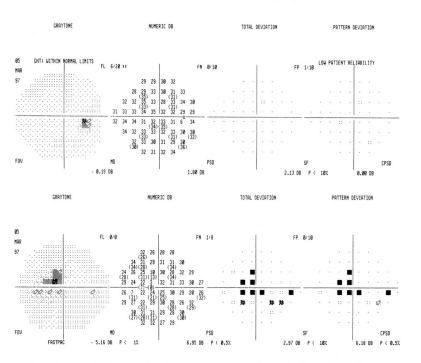

Figure 5.5 Humphrey perimeter visual field assessment: toxoplasmosis. There is a defined central area of left visual field loss extending to the blind spot producing a caecocentral scotoma. The right central visual field is normal.

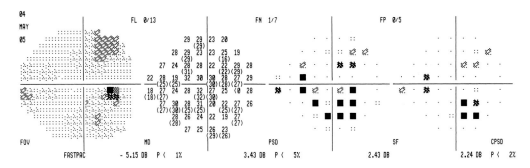

Figure 5.6 Humphrey perimeter visual field assessment: retinopathy. Visual field loss is documented that does not conform to a pattern.

References

Ballantyne AJ (1946) The nerve fibre pattern of the human retina. *Transactions of the Ophthalmic Societies of the UK*, **66**: 179

Heijl A, Patella VM (2002) *The Field Analyzer Primer. Essential Perimetry*, 3rd edn. Dublin, CA, Carl Zeiss Meditec

Jabs DA (1996) Acquired immunodeficiency syndrome and the eye. *Archives of Ophthalmology*, **114**: 863

Radius RL, Anderson DL (1979) The course of axons through the retina and optic nerve head. *Archives of Ophthalmology*, **97**: 1154

Vrabec F (1966) The temporal raphe of the human retina. *American Journal of Ophthalmology*, **62**: 926

Further reading

Adler FH, Kaufman PL (eds) (2002)*Adler's Physiology of the Eye. Clinical Application*, 10th edn. St Louis, Mosby

Birchall CH, Harrisw GS, Drance SM, Gegg IS (1976) Visual field changes in branch retinal vein occlusion. *Archives of Ophthalmology*, **94**: 747

Hayreh SS (1963) The central artery of the retina. *British Journal of Ophthalmology*, **47**: 651

Kanski J (2003) *Clinical Opthalmology. A Systematic Approach*, 5th edn. London, Butterworth Heinemann

Kanski J (2004) *Clinical Opthalmology. A Synopsis*. London, Butterworth Heinmann/Elsevier Science

Mangat HS (1995) Retinal artery occlusion. *Survey of Ophthalmology*, **40**: 145

Minckler DS (1980) The organization of nerve fibre bundles in the primate optic nerve head. *Archives of Ophthalmology*, **98**: 1630

Olver J, Cassidy L (2005) *Opthalmology at a Glance*. Oxford, Blackwell Publishing

Snell RS, Lemp MA (1998) *Clinical Anatomy of the Eye*, 2nd edn. Oxford, Blackwell Publishing

Tripathi RC, Tripathi BJ (1970) Anatomy of the human eye, orbit and adnexa. In: *The Eye*, 3rd edn (ed. H Davson). London, Academic Press

Trobe JD, Bergsma DR (1975) Atypical retinitis pigmentosa masquerading as nerve fiber bundle lesion. *American Journal of Ophthalmology*, **79**: 681

Chapter 6
Optic nerve

Anatomy*

The optic nerve consists of axons of retinal ganglion cells and extends from the optic disc to the optic chiasm. It can be divided into four portions:

(1) Intraorbital
(2) Orbital
(3) Intracanalicular
(4) Intracranial.

The intraorbital portion of the optic nerve includes the optic disc and the portion of the optic nerve within the posterior scleral foramen. The optic disc is the commencement of the optic nerve. It is approximately 1.5 mm in diameter and is significantly paler in colour than the surrounding retina. The optic disc is located about 3 mm nasal to and about 0.8 mm above the fovea. It is composed of axons of ganglion cells that leave the eye through the lamina cribrosa. The optic disc is oval in shape and the optic cup is a funnel-shaped depression within the disc where the central retina vessels enter and leave the eye. There are no ganglion cell axons in the optic cup (see Fig. 5.1). The layers of the retina and choroid terminate at the edge of the optic disc, and the absence of photoreceptors in this area explains the blind spot of the visual field. Posterior to the optic disc, the nerve fibres become myelinated.

The orbital portion of the optic nerve has an 'S' shaped curve to permit movement of the eye. It is covered with a dense dural sheath, an arachnoid sheath and pia mater. These extend from the optic foramen to the eye, where the dura mater and arachnoid sheaths blend with the sclera. The central core of the orbital optic nerve consists predominantly of the papillomacular bundle, which contains the nerve fibres that

---

*This anatomy section is intended as a brief description only. If required, further detail should be sought from appropriate textbooks – see Further reading. The anatomy and pathology sections, in combination, provide a background to the part of the visual pathway covered in this chapter so that the relevant visual field defects can be considered and interpreted appropriately.

subserve the cone system of the fovea, and also peripheral nasal and temporal retinal nerve fibres.

The intracanalicular portion of the optic nerve passes through the optic foramen. At the anterior portion of the optic foramen, the dural sheath covering the nerve divides so that one portion continues as the periosteum of the orbit. The other portion continues as the dural sheath of the optic nerve. In the optic foramen, the dural sheath is adherent to bone, arachnoid and pia mater, so that the nerve is firmly fixed in this position.

The intracranial portion passes medially from the optic canal to form the optic chiasm with the contralateral optic nerve.

The arrangement of fibres in the optic disc and optic nerve corresponds generally to the distribution of fibres in the retina (Anderson 1970; Radius & Anderson 1979a,b). Superior retinal fibres are represented in the superior part of the optic nerve head, inferior fibres are below, and the nasal and temporal fibres are on their respective sides. The papillomacular bundle is a sector shaped structure occupying approximately one-third of the optic disc temporally adjacent to the central blood vessels. This bundle of central retinal nerve fibres moves centrally within the optic nerve as it moves towards the optic chiasm. Therefore, more posteriorly in the orbit, the macular fibres lie in the centre of the nerve. Superior and inferior macular fibres retain their relative positions throughout the nerve while crossed (central temporal visual field) macular fibres lie nasal to the uncrossed (central nasal visual field) fibres. The gradual movement of the macular fibres to the centre of the nerve allows the peripheral superior and inferior retinal nerve fibres to come together.

The optic nerve is supplied by branches of blood vessels from a number of sources: the central retinal vessels and branches (ophthalmic artery), scleral vessels (circle of Zinn–Haller), choroidal vessels and pial vessels (from adjacent branches of the internal carotid artery) (Francois & Neetans 1954, 1963; Francois *et al.* 1955; Cioffi & van Buskirk 1994; Chou *et al.* 1995).

Pathology*

Congenital abnormalities

Congenital anomalies include aplasia and hypoplasia of the optic nerve, coloboma, optic atrophy, optic pit and tilted disc. Recognition and diagnosis of congenital optic disc anomalies are important because such anomalies are common, differential diagnosis from papilloedema is imperative, they may give rise to visual field defects, they may be associated with other central nervous system abnormalities and may cause significant central visual problems due to macular involvement.

---

*This pathology section is provided as a summary of possible disease processes but by its nature cannot be all inclusive. The reader is directed towards other appropriate textbooks for further detail – see Further reading.

Coloboma

Coloboma results from an incomplete closure of foetal tissue. The disc contains a very large excavation which is usually situated inferiorly, so that normal disc tissue is confined to a small superior wedge (Colour Plate 6.1). The coloboma itself is surrounded by an elevated annulus of chorioretinal pigmentary disturbance. A common association is a non-rhegmatogenous retinal detachment.

Drusen (hyaline bodies)

Drusen are deposits of a hyaline-like calcific material (Tso 1981) within the tissue of the optic nerve head (Colour Plate 6.2). Drusen may not be visible, particularly if buried within the tissue of the optic disc.

Morning glory syndrome

This very rare dysplastic coloboma of the optic disc resembles the morning glory flower. The optic nerve head appears enlarged and excavated (Colour Plate 6.3) and contains persistent hyaloid remnants within its base (Pollock 1987; Eustis *et al.* 1994). The blood vessels emerge from the rim of the excavation in a radial pattern similar to the spokes of a wheel.

Myelinated nerve fibres

Myelinated nerve fibres are a common congenital abnormality which may be mistaken for disc oedema. Normally, myelination of the anterior visual system begins at the lateral geniculate body during gestation and proceeds towards the eyes, stopping at the lamina cribrosa. Further intraocular myelination may follow several patterns, the most common being that of extensive myelination beginning at the disc and extending towards the retinal periphery. The myelinated nerve fibres follow the pattern of the normal nerve fibre layers and extend as irregular feather-shaped patterns which may or may not obscure the retinal vessels (Colour Plate 6.4). Although myelination is most frequently seen adjacent to the optic disc, patches of peripheral myelination may also occur.

Optic disc pit

This relatively common condition consists of a round or oval pit which appears darker than the surrounding disc tissue (Brown *et al.* 1980). The location is most frequently inferotemporal on the optic disc (Colour Plate 6.5). About 50% of eyes with congenital optic pits develop oedema or a serous detachment of the macula. This can mimic central serous chorioretinopathy.

Optic nerve hypoplasia

Optic nerve hypoplasia may be complete or partial (Buchanan & Hoyt 1981). If present, it is bilateral in at least 50% of cases. The typical appearance of optic nerve hypoplasia is that of a small grey optic disc surrounded by a yellow halo of hypopigmentation (Lambert *et al.* 1987). The lack of pigmentation relates to a concentric choroidal and retinal pigment epithelial abnormality. This appearance is referred to as the double ring sign. Despite the small optic disc, the retinal blood vessels emerging from it are of normal calibre.

Tilted disc

The presence of a congenital tilted optic disc is fairly common, usually bilateral (Colour Plate 6.6) and the condition is due to the optic nerve entering the globe at an oblique angle (Guiffre 1986). The disc has an exaggerated oval appearance with the vertical axis directed obliquely so that its upper temporal portion lies anterior to the lower margin. This appearance may be mistaken for papilloedema. Eyes with tilted discs frequently have an inferior crescent, situs inversus of the retinal blood vessels, myopia, a moderate degree of oblique astigmatism and hypopigmentation involving the inferonasal aspect of the retina (Brazitikos *et al.* 1990).

Acquired abnormalities

Compression

Compressive lesions may be posterior to the globe or within the optic nerve itself.

Masses of the optic disc

These include congenital elevations, epipapillary astrocytomas, acquired disc swelling, vascular hamartomas (capillary and cavernous haemangiomas), melanocytomas, retinoblastomas, metastatic carcinoma, lymphoblastic and myeloblastic leukaemic infiltrates and sarcoid granulomas.

Thyroid eye disease

This can cause visual loss due to orbital congestion (Fig. 6.1). Extraocular muscles are enlarged by infiltration and the optic nerves are encroached on by swollen muscles at the tight orbital apex where it is likely that the optic nerves are compressed (Gasser & Flammer 1986).

Tumours

Tumours are often primary, with spread along the optic nerve between the orbit and cranial cavity. Optic nerve tumours include gliomas and meningiomas. Compression of the optic chiasm is a frequent mode of presentation in addition to involvement of the optic nerve. Tumours arising at the lateral portion of the sphenoid bone may extend into the orbit and cause proptosis in addition to optic nerve compression.

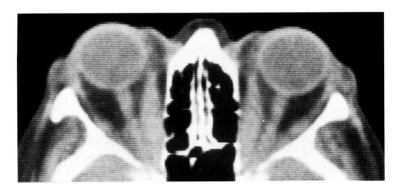

Figure 6.1 Crowded orbital apex in thyroid eye disease. Neuroimaging reveals there is increased bulk of extraocular muscles that compress the optic nerve at the apex of the orbit. Such compressive optic neuropathy is a medial ophthalmic emergency requiring decompression of the orbital volume.

Glioma typically affects children; it is associated commonly with neurofibromatosis and usually involves the optic canal.

Meningiomas are invasive tumours which typically affect middle aged women. Ocular features are related to the location of the tumours. Optic nerve sheath meningiomas (Colour Plate 6.7 and Fig. 6.2a) usually arise from meningothelial cells of the arachnoid and are initially confined by the surrounding dura.

Neurofibroma is composed mainly of proliferations of Schwann cells within the neural sheaths. Plexiform neurofibromas typically occur in patients with neurofibromatosis. Complete surgical removal is extremely difficult.

Paranasal sinus disease can cause visual loss, proptosis, diplopia or headache.

Glaucoma

Intraocular pressure is determined by the balance between production of aqueous fluid by the ciliary body and drainage of aqueous fluid via the trabecular meshwork. It has a mean value of 16 mmHg which rises in the older population. Interference with blood flow or axonal transport at the superior and inferior poles of the optic disc, in particular due to pressure differentials at the optic disc, results in glaucoma with loss of retinal ganglion cells.

There is a high risk of developing glaucoma in patients with intraocular pressure greater than 24 mmHg, a strong family history, previous or current treatment with topical or systemic steroids, conditions that affect the filtration angle such as pigment dispersion syndrome and uveitis, and congenital malformations of the filtration angle. The classical feature of damage to the optic nerve in glaucoma is cupping of the optic disc (Colour Plate 6.8). The increased cup : disc ratio is due to decreased neural rim tissue.

Ocular hypertension

This is associated with an intraocular pressure greater than 21 mmHg with normal visual fields and optic discs.

Normal tension glaucoma

This has a normal range intraocular pressure, but with abnormal visual fields and optic discs. Normal low tension glaucoma may be associated with vasospastic diseases such as migraine and Raynaud's phenomenon.

Primary open angle glaucoma

This has an insidious onset. The relationship between the iris root, the trabecular meshwork and the cornea is normal. The drainage resistance in the trabecular meshwork may be increased as a result of a block within the trabecular tissue, such as progressive increase in the collagen content of the trabecular fibres, resulting in narrowing of the meshwork pores.

Secondary open angle glaucoma

In secondary open angle glaucoma the trabecular meshwork is blocked, for example by haemorrhage following trauma, inflammatory cells or material produced by the epithelium of the lens, iris and ciliary body.

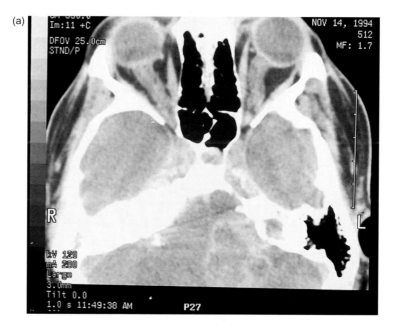

Figure 6.2 Bilateral optic nerve meningioma. (a) Note the thickened appearance of the optic nerves on this scan and also the large sphenoid wing meningioma in the middle cranial fossa; additional meningiomas were scattered in the brain parenchyma. (b,c) On visual field assessment, progressive visual field loss is seen over time: Goldmann fields at first assessment show a normal left peripheral visual field with enlarged blind spot and marked temporal visual field loss of the right eye; follow-up visual fields using Humphrey automated perimetry for the left eye demonstrate progression to temporal and inferior nasal visual field involvement resulting in generalised constriction with loss of the central area also. This is the same patient as Colour Plate 6.7.

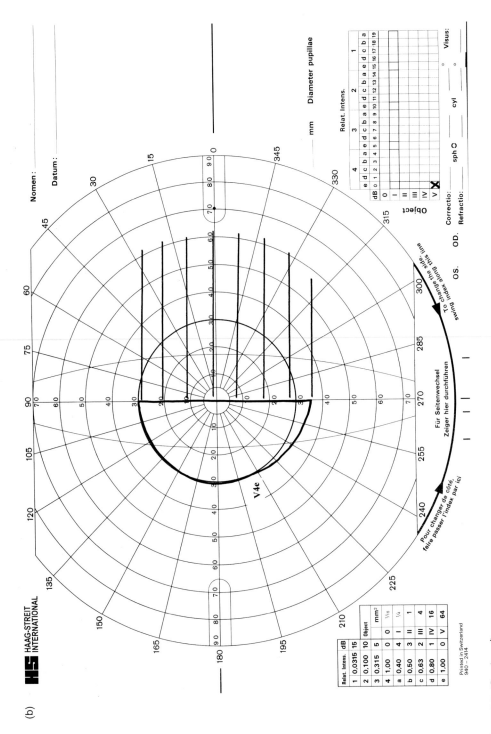

(b)

Figure 6.2 (Continued)

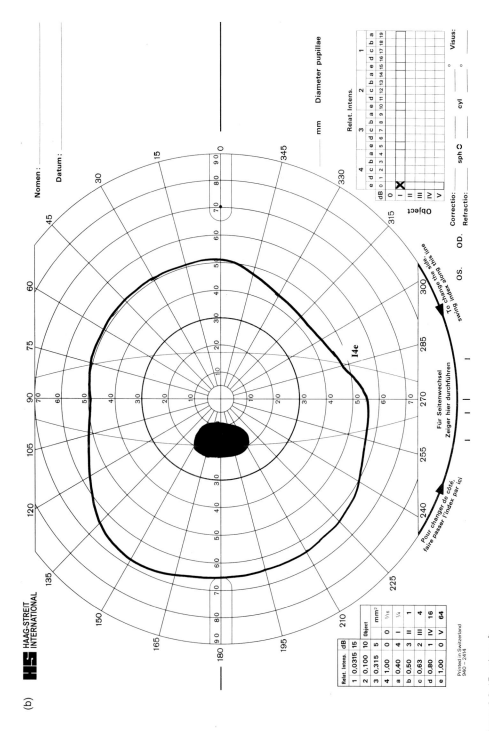

Figure 6.2 (Continued)

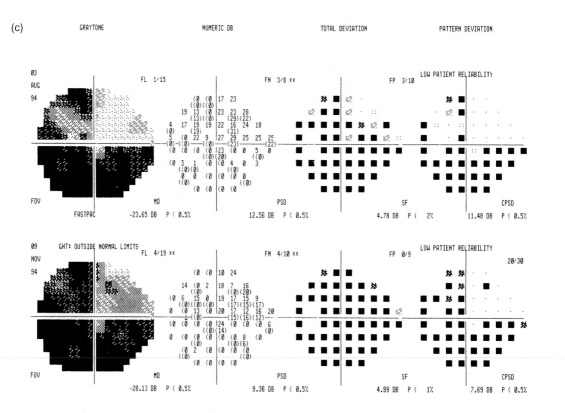

Figure 6.2 (Continued)

Primary closed angle glaucoma

The iris root is displaced forward, blocking the trabecular meshwork and obstructing the outflow. This generally occurs with age where the iris is displaced anteriorly by an enlarging lens resulting in a shallower anterior chamber. As the angles become narrower, pressure builds up behind the iris and pushes the peripheral iris towards the trabecular meshwork thus obstructing outflow.

Secondary closed angle glaucoma

This is most commonly caused by inflammatory conditions in which fibrin initiates adhesion formation between the peripheral iris and the trabecular meshwork, or the iris and lens, resulting in obstruction to flow of aqueous fluid in the angle or at the pupil.

Hereditary abnormalities
Leber's optic neuropathy

A rare hereditary disorder primarily affecting healthy young men, it has autosomal recessive inheritance.

Inflammatory neuropathy

Optic or retrobulbar neuritis

This is an inflammatory or demyelinating disorder of the optic nerve (Colour Plate 6.9). It may be idiopathic or due to a variety of causes such as demyelination, which is a common manifestation of multiple sclerosis. Optic neuritis is the presenting sign in 25% of patients with multiple sclerosis and occurs during the course of established disease in about 70%. Optic neuritis may also occur after viral illness, following granulomatous inflammation, or as an associated infection of the meninges, sinuses or orbit. The typical episode involves one eye only, although in children especially it is not unusual for bilateral neuritis to follow viral illness.

Optic papillitis

This condition is common in children. The inflammation involves the intraocular portion of the optic nerve, giving rise to swelling of the optic nerve head with obliteration of the physiological cup and inflammatory cells in the vitreous.

Oedema

Papilloedema and pseudopapilloedema are forms of oedema (swelling) of the optic disc. Papilloedema is associated with raised intracranial pressure. The cerebrospinal fluid is formed by the choroid plexus in both lateral ventricles and in the third ventricle, from where it flows through the aqueduct of Sylvius to the fourth ventricle. The cerebrospinal fluid partly flows around the spinal cord and the remainder bathes the cerebral hemispheres. It is finally absorbed into the cerebral venous drainage system through the arachnoid villi along the venous sinuses.

Swelling of the optic disc may be unilateral or bilateral and may be congenital (pseudopapilloedema), due to true papilloedema with raised intracranial pressure, swelling with associated local ocular diseases (uveitis, central retinal vein occlusion, optic neuritis), primary nerve head tumours and optic nerve compression.

Conditions resulting in papilloedema include intracranial mass, subdural haematoma, epidural haematoma, brain abscess, arterivenous malformations, subarachnoid haemorrhage, trauma, meningitis, encephalitis, spinal cord tumours, craniostenosis and idiopathic intracranial hypertension.

When the disc is swollen, its margin is indistinct and it may appear elevated. The central cup region of the disc may be obliterated by swollen tissue; the retinal venules may be dilated and tortuous, and venous pulsation is absent. Axoplasmic transport along the retinal nerve fibres in the optic disc and optic nerve is delayed by the raised intracranial pressure. Fluid backs into the retinal tissues surrounding the disc producing the swelling. Stages of papilloedema include early, acute, chronic and vintage (Colour Plates 6.10 to 6.13). Secondary vascular changes may eventually produce a secondary optic atrophy (Colour Plate 6.14).

Optic atrophy

A normal optic disc should be pink with a clearly defined edge. In optic atrophy there is stark pallor of the disc (Colour Plate 6.14). Causes of optic atrophy include glaucoma, papilloedema, ischaemia, drug toxicity, demyelination, trauma, compression of the anterior visual pathway, viral infections and retinal dystrophy.

Toxic optic neuropathies

Toxic amblyopia

This condition affects heavy drinkers and pipe smokers who have a diet deficient in protein and B vitamins (Foulds *et al.* 1970).

Drug induced optic neuropathy

May occur with either prescribed or non-prescribed medications. Ethambutol used for the treatment of tuberculosis produces optic neuropathy if used in high doses. Other drugs which may affect the optic nerve include chloramphenicol, isoniazid and streptomycin.

Vascular abnormalities

Disruption of blood supply to the optic nerve such as with thrombus or atherosclerosis results in ischaemic optic neuropathy.

Aneurysm

As the intracranial portion of the optic nerve ascends from the optic canal to the optic chiasm it lies immediately above the initial supracavernous segment of the internal carotid artery. Ectatic dilation of this segment of the internal carotid artery may compress the optic nerve from below, compressing it against the unyielding periforaminal dura, anterior clinoid and anterior cerebral artery.

Anterior ischaemic optic neuropathy

This is a relatively common cause of severe visual loss in the middle aged and elderly. The pathology involves a segmental or generalised infarction of the anterior part of the optic nerve caused by occlusion of the short posterior ciliary arteries. This may be secondary to atherosclerosis, giant cell arteritis, collagen vascular disorders (e.g. systemic lupus erythematosis), or emboli such as with papilloedema, malignant hypertension or migraine.

Non-arteritic anterior ischaemic optic neuropathy occurs as an isolated event in individuals between the ages of 45 and 65 years who are otherwise healthy or who have hypertension as the only sign of systemic vascular disease.

Arteritic anterior ischaemic optic neuropathy is caused by **giant cell arteritis**, is a necrotising systemic vasculitis with a predilection for the cranial arteries. Patients are often unwell with fatigue, weight loss and severe focal hemicranial headache. Without immediate treatment, irreversible bilateral visual loss may occur. The most common vasculitis responsible for neuro-ophthalmic symptoms and signs is cranial arteritis, and the frequent presentation is a usually severe form of ischaemic optic neuropathy occurring in an older age group and usually with devastating visual loss.

Associated signs and symptoms*

An optic nerve lesion not only diminishes visual acuity and produces a visual field defect, but it also impairs three other aspects of optic nerve function: the afferent pupillary pathways, colour vision and contrast sensitivity. Patients may complain of transient visual obscurations and amaurosis fugax, reduced visual acuity and reduced colour vision.

Congenital anomalous discs can be associated with loss of visual acuity or visual field of varying degree. Hypoplastic discs are associated with poor acuity, field defect and small discs. Acquired optic nerve disease is usually represented by acute or subacute progressive dimming of central vision.

Anterior segment appearance

The eye in acute angle closure glaucoma appears injected with a hazy oedematous cornea and an oval, non-reactive mid-dilated pupil.

Colour vision

Optic nerve disease is associated with colour loss, often in the red–green axis (Schneck & Haegerstrom-Portnoy 1997; Flanagan & Zele 2004). Visual function in optic neuritis is depressed over the entire field, but most markedly involves the central 20 degrees with variable diminution of colour vision.

Contrast sensitivity

Visual function in optic neuritis is depressed over the entire field with variable diminution of contrast sensitivity.

Fundus appearance

On examination of the optic disc in glaucoma, cupping may be recognised. This should be graded in comparison to the fellow eye. Optic disc pallor or disc swelling

---

*This section on associated signs and symptoms is provided so that the practitioner is aware of additional information that can be considered in conjunction with the visual field defect to aid differential diagnosis and localisation of pathology.

may be observed in optic nerve tumours. Patients may have retinochoroidal striae. Disc oedema and flame shaped haemorrhages may be seen on fundus examination in patients with vascular abnormalities and optic disc papilloedema.

Patients with optic neuropathy present with sudden loss of vision in the affected eye and the disc is usually pale and swollen. Peri-disc splinter haemorrhages are often seen.

The appearance of disc pallor in optic atrophy depends on the nature of the offending lesion, the time interval, the degree of axonal attrition and the distance of the lesion from the optic nerve head.

Ocular appearance

Optic nerve tumours may present with unilateral proptosis and visual impairment. Strabismus may also be noted. As meningiomas grow within the dural sheath, they cause a splinting of the optic nerve which impairs ocular movements, especially on upgaze. Later, as the tumour extends through the dura to form an enlarging mass within the muscle cone, it results in proptosis. Patients may have increasing hyperopia.

Patients with optic neuritis may have an impairment of binocular depth perception.

Pupil abnormalities

Division of one nerve results in blindness of that eye and a pupil which does not react directly to light but does consensually, because the motor part of the reflex pathway is intact. The affected pupil will react to convergence.

Visual perception

Acute angle closure glaucoma patients present with severe ocular and periorbital pain. Pain in angle closure glaucoma is nauseating ocular pain.

Tenderness of the globe and deep orbital or brow pain, especially with eye movements, may precede or coincide with visual impairment in cases of retrobulbar neuritis. Abrupt onset of monocular visual dysfunction in the age group up to the fifth decade, with a normal appearing optic disc, is highly suggestive of retrobulbar neuritis, especially if accompanied by a dull orbital pain or discomfort of the globe itself. Patients may have an increase in visual deficit with exercise (Uhthoffs symptom).

Patients experience brief transient loss of vision in papilloedema (transient visual obscurations) (Sadun *et al.* 1984).

There is a strong link between ischaemic optic neuropathy and giant cell temporal arteritis. Temporal artery or scalp tenderness indicates giant cell arteritis.

Visual acuity

Myelinated nerve fibres can be associated with poor vision.

Acute angle closure glaucoma patients present with reduced vision. Vision is obscured by halos around light sources.

Optic neuritis (inflammation) is associated with relatively acute impairment of vision, progressing rapidly for hours or days. Visual function usually reaches its lowest level by 1–2 weeks after onset. Visual function is depressed over the entire field but most markedly involves the central 20 degrees with variable diminution of acuity, colour sense and contrast sensitivity.

Central loss of vision is uncommon in papilloedema until the late stages of optic disc swelling.

Retrobulbar disease producing abrupt to subacute loss in the elderly includes cranial arteritis and meningeal metastases. Slowly progressive monocular visual loss over many months typifies chronic tumoral compression of the optic nerve in its prechiasmal portion. Meningiomas present with a slowly progressive impairment of vision in one eye from optic nerve compression. Paranasal sinus visual loss is usually monocular and slowly progressive.

Vascular lesions typically result in sudden onset of complete or partial visual loss. In the older age group, the single most common optic nerve disease that presents as apoplectic loss of vision is ischaemic infarct of the disc – anterior ischaemic optic neuropathy. Ischaemic optic neuropathy is associated with sudden painless loss of vision in one eye with little improvement over time. Patients with aneurysms may have insidious or rapid visual loss.

Visual field defects

The most frequent visual field defect in optic nerve disease is the central scotoma. Typically, monocular visual field deficits are the rule in optic nerve disease unless both optic nerves are involved. Hereditary atrophies and toxic/nutritional neuropathies are bilateral, but they may be asymmetric.

It is estimated that about 30% of nerve fibres in the optic nerve must be damaged before a reproducible visual field defect becomes apparent (Kerrigan-Baumrind *et al.* 2000). Visual field defects also include central depression and nerve fibre bundle defects. Altitudinal defects are more usually vascular in origin. Optic disc disease typically shows inferior nasal predilection. Insidious bilateral central or caecocentral scotomas are hallmarks of intrinsic optic nerve disease resulting from nutritional deficiencies, intake of toxins or hereditary atrophies. Rarely, demyelination disease runs such a slowly progressive course.

When a central field defect is found in one eye, careful search of the temporal field of the contralateral eye is mandatory to rule out the possibility of junctional compression (optic nerve and optic chiasm). Most prechiasmal optic neuropathies are due to inflammatory or vascular disease, whereas practically all optic chiasm syndromes are due to pituitary adenomas, other neoplasms or aneurysm compression.

Congenital abnormalities

Coloboma

Eyes with colobomas often have decreased vision and superior visual field defects. Visual field defects do not always reflect the appearance of the coloboma. They may resemble glaucoma defects with dense nerve fibre bundle defects and nasal depression.

Drusen

These may produce extensive and slowly progressive visual field defects of which nerve fibre bundle defects are common. Visual field defects are due to the drusen pressing on nerve fibres (Gutteridge & Cockburn 1981; Roh *et al.* 1998). Drusen of the nerve head often have irregular enlargement of blind spots (Fig. 6.3). Nerve fibre bundle defects commonly course inferonasally. Irregular general peripheral contraction and wedge defects are also seen.

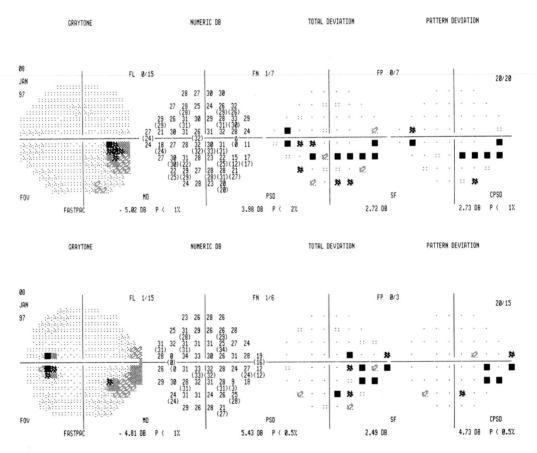

Figure 6.3 Humphrey perimeter visual field assessment: optic disc drusen. Enlarged blind spots are documented with nasal inferior visual field loss of the right eye.

Myelinated nerve fibres

Generally, visual acuity is normal; however, the blind spot may be enlarged. Visual field involvement can vary substantially. The visual field loss corresponds to the anatomic location of the myelinated nerve fibres and to their density and thickness (Fig. 6.4).

Optic disc pit

With optic disc pits the most common visual field defects relate to nerve fibre bundle involvement. There may be macular involvement of the visual field as the pit may cause a subretinal oedema in the macula, resulting in a central scotoma.

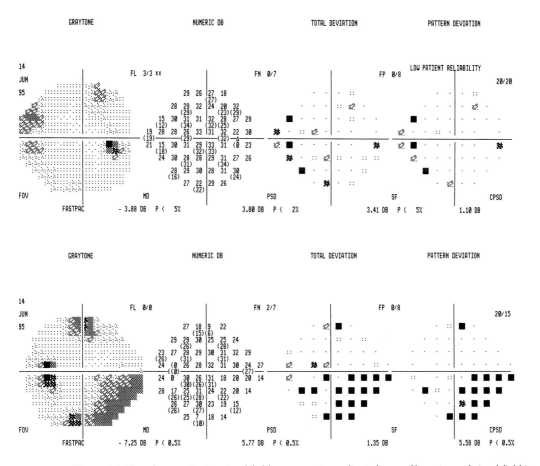

Figure 6.4 Humphrey perimeter visual field assessment: myelinated nerve fibres. Loss of visual field is dependent on the extent of nerve fibre myelination and involvement of the nerve fibre layer. Visual field loss can vary considerably. These visual fields show enlarged blind spots with predominantly nasal visual field involvement.

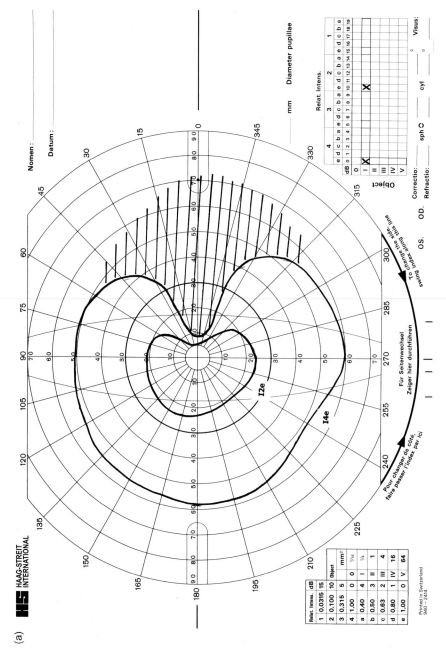

Figure 6.5 Goldmann and Humphrey perimeter visual field assessment: optic nerve hypoplasia. The optic disc may be completely under-developed (aplasia) or partially under-developed (hypoplasia). Where there is hypoplasia of an area of the optic disc, visual field loss relates specifically to this area. There is a temporal sector defect extending to the optic disc. This is more apparent on Goldmann (a) peripheral visual field assessment than Humphrey (b) central visual field assessment. There is also nasal inferior visual field loss relating to co-existent papilloedema.

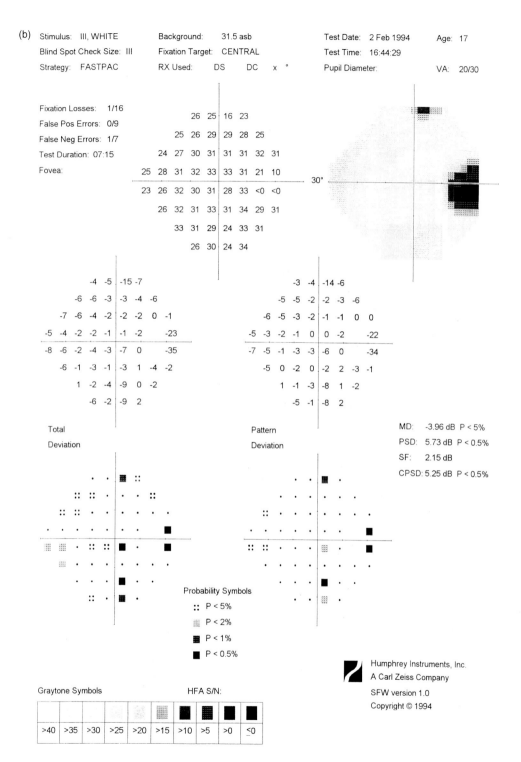

(b)

Stimulus: III, WHITE	Background: 31.5 asb	Test Date: 2 Feb 1994	Age: 17
Blind Spot Check Size: III	Fixation Target: CENTRAL	Test Time: 16:44:29	
Strategy: FASTPAC	RX Used: DS DC x °	Pupil Diameter:	VA: 20/30

Fixation Losses: 1/16
False Pos Errors: 0/9
False Neg Errors: 1/7
Test Duration: 07:15
Fovea:

```
                26  25 | 16  23
            25  26  29 | 29  28  25
        24  27  30  31 | 31  31  32  31
    25  28  31  32  33 | 33  31  21  10
    23  26  32  30  31 | 28  33  <0  <0        30°
        26  32  31  33 | 31  34  29  31
            33  31  29 | 24  33  31
                26  30 | 24  34
```

Total Deviation

```
            -4  -5 | -15  -7
        -6  -6  -3 | -3  -4  -6
    -7  -6  -4  -2 | -2  -2   0  -1
 -5 -4  -2  -2  -1 | -1  -2      -23
 -8 -6  -2  -4  -3 | -7   0      -35
    -6  -1  -3  -1 | -3   1  -4  -2
         1  -2  -4 | -9   0  -2
            -6  -2 | -9   2
```

Pattern Deviation

```
            -3  -4 | -14  -6
        -5  -5  -2 | -2  -3  -6
    -6  -5  -3  -2 | -1  -1   0   0
 -5 -3  -2  -1   0 |  0  -2      -22
 -7 -5  -1  -3  -3 | -6   0      -34
    -5   0  -2   0 | -2   2  -3  -1
         1  -1  -3 | -8   1  -2
            -5  -1 | -8   2
```

MD: -3.96 dB P < 5%
PSD: 5.73 dB P < 0.5%
SF: 2.15 dB
CPSD: 5.25 dB P < 0.5%

Probability Symbols

∷ P < 5%
▦ P < 2%
▩ P < 1%
■ P < 0.5%

Humphrey Instruments, Inc.
A Carl Zeiss Company
SFW version 1.0
Copyright © 1994

Graytone Symbols   HFA S/N:

>40	>35	>30	>25	>20	>15	>10	>5	>0	≤0

Figure 6.5 (Continued)

Optic nerve hypoplasia

If severe, optic nerve hypoplasia can result in marked impairment of visual acuity and an afferent pupillary conduction defect. Visual field examination may show nasal or temporal defects (Fig. 6.5), small arcuate defects, altitudinal hemianopias and coecocentral scotomas. Visual field defects vary from minimal involvement to total blindness and may be bilateral.

Tilted disc

Tilted optic discs may produce an upper temporal field defect which can possibly be mistaken for optic chiasm compression (Brazitikos *et al.* 1990).

Acquired abnormalities

Glaucoma

Open angle glaucoma is the most common form of optic nerve pathology. Visual field assessment is used to document the extent and change in visual field over time. It is of diagnostic and therapeutic importance, particularly for primary open angle glaucoma, as these cases are initially asymptomatic.

Stages of glaucomatous visual field defects have been proposed:

(1) Only relative visual field defects
(2) Absolute visual field defects, but not yet in connection with the blind spot
(3) Absolute arcuate visual field defects in connection with the blind spot, producing a nasal step
(4) Extensive absolute visual field defects with central island remaining
(5) Visual field defects involving the centre but with an island of vision remaining temporally.

The classic features of glaucoma are loss in the dense superior and inferior arcuate retinal nerve fibre bundles and prolonged sparing of the central papillomacular area that subserves visual acuity (Drance 1972; Hart & Becker 1982). Therefore with visual field loss in the caecocentral area, a neurologic lesion may be suspected. Visual field defects that preferentially involve the nasal field but without a hemianopic character (aligned on the vertical meridian) are most likely to be due to glaucoma.

Most visual field defects occur within the central 30 degrees of visual field, although the peripheral field is frequently involved (Stewart & Schields 1991). Generalised loss of visual field occurs with depression of threshold sensitivity and constriction of peripheral isopters. Focal loss of visual field is typical, and visual field defects follow retinal nerve fibre layer involvement (Fig. 6.6). Traditionally, focal loss includes paracentral scotomas (Fig. 6.7), arcuates (Fig. 6.8) and nasal steps (Fig. 6.9), most of which are found in the central 30 degrees of the visual field. Paracentral defects usually occur in the arcuate area between 10 and 20 degrees of eccentricity. Arcuate defects indicate a more advanced state.

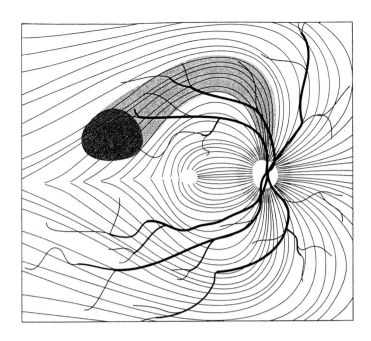

Figure 6.6 Representation of nerve fibre bundle loss. With focal optic disc pathology the damaged retinal nerve fibres project in an arcuate pattern and are approximately the same length. Reproduced with permission (Heijl & Patella 2002)

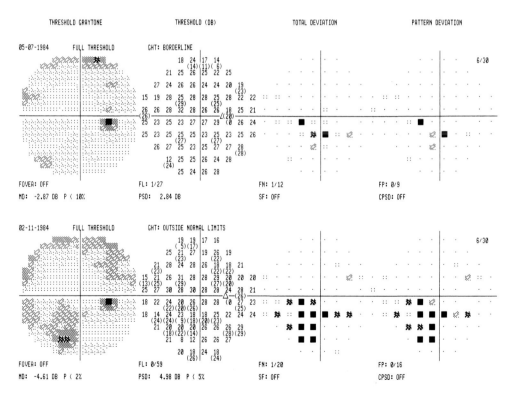

Figure 6.7 Humphrey perimeter visual field assessment: paracentral scotomas (glaucoma). The right eye shows paracentral scotomatous visual field loss with early arcuate visual field deficit.

Nasal step is a difference in sensitivity above and below the horizontal meridian in the nasal field. Overall depression of the visual field indicates a diffuse loss of nerve fibres throughout the optic nerve. Eventually global constriction occurs, but with preservation of the central macular visual field until late in the course of the disease.

Visual field defects can develop very slowly and therefore appear quite stable for a considerable period of time (Fig. 6.8). As a result, it is important for appropriate

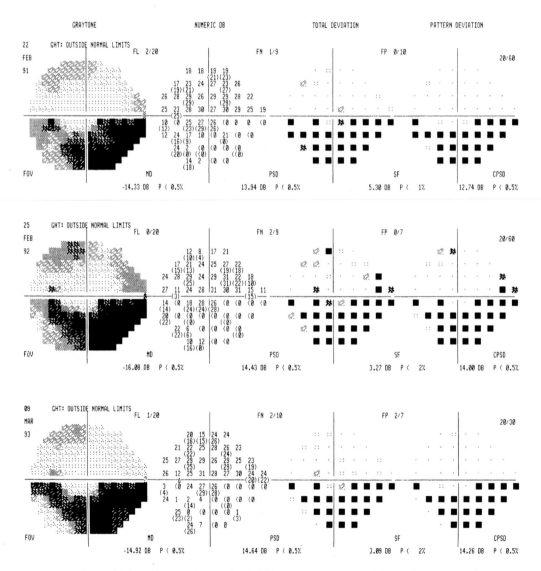

Figure 6.8 Humphrey perimeter visual field assessment: arcuate defects (glaucoma). A dense superior arcuate defect is present in the right eye with a dense inferior arcuate of the left eye. These defects are relatively stable over time.

monitoring procedures to be in place. Visual field defects can also develop quite aggressively, rendering the patient visually disabled within a relatively short period of time. Visual loss can develop simultaneously in both eyes (Figs 6.9 and 6.10) or asymmetrically (Fig. 6.11) with similar or dissimilar patterns of visual field loss (Fig. 6.12). Where dissimilar patterns of visual field loss occur, the patients are generally not as aware of the severity of their visual loss as either eye will compensate for the other to a certain extent.

Visual field loss is frequently asymmetrical; hence the glaucoma hemifield test is used in automated perimetry (Asman & Heijl 1991; Katz *et al.* 1996).

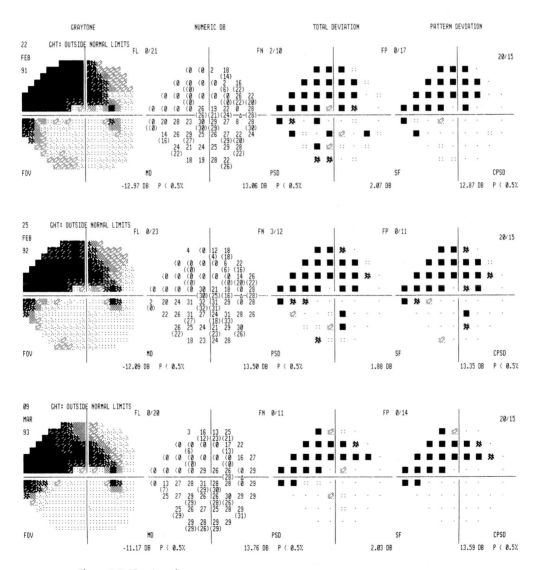

Figure 6.8 (Continued)

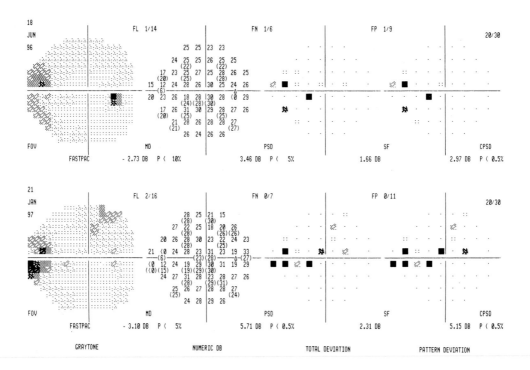

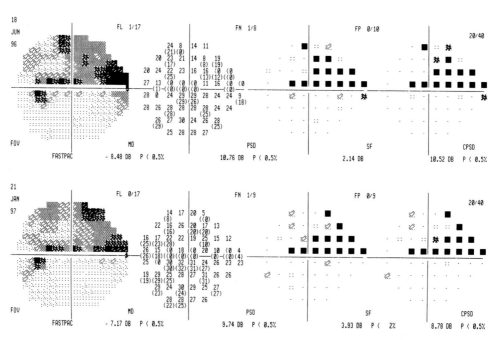

Figure 6.9 Humphrey perimeter visual field assessment: nasal steps (glaucoma). A nasal step is present in the right eye with further development over a period of time. A nasal step and superior arcuate defect are present in the left eye.

Inflammation

Optic or retrobulbar neuritis may result in visual field impairment ranging from quite mild to severe. The visual field findings of optic and retrobulbar neuritis typically include varieties of central and caecocentral scotomas (Figs 6.13 and 6.14) but also may show nerve fibre bundle (Fig. 6.15) and altitudinal defects, general constriction (Fig. 6.16) and reduced sensitivity across the central visual field (Fig. 6.17). Typically, the main visual field loss is confined to the affected eye. However, it is not unusual to find subtle defects in the other eye (Figs 6.14 and 6.17) and optic or retrobulbar neuritis may also occur as a quite definite bilateral involvement (Figs 6.17, 6.18 and 6.19). Atypical visual field results may show a combination of a central or caecocentral scotoma with other visual field impairment such as nasal field loss (Fig. 6.20) and paracentral scotomas (Fig. 6.18). In most cases, visual function begins to improve in the second or third week (Fig. 6.13).

Oedema

Visual field involvement with optic disc oedema is typically bilateral, but can be symmetrical or asymmetrical. Papilloedema stages include early, acute, chronic, vintage and atrophic. Early papilloedema is associated with normal visual acuity, visual fields (apart from an enlarged blind spot; Fig. 6.21) and pupillary functions. Acute papilloedema shows multiple fundus haemorrhages and increased swelling of the optic disc, and therefore is more prone to nerve fibre bundle defects in the visual field (Fig. 6.22).

With persistent papilloedema over a number of weeks or months, chronic papilloedema is seen and the nerve fibre bundle involvement results in progressive visual field loss in the form of paracentral scotomas, arcuate defects and peripheral constriction of the visual field (Figs 6.23 and 6.24). Vintage papilloedema which has been present for a considerable period of time is associated with severe constriction of the visual field. The central visual field is relatively spared until involved with vintage severe papilloedema or optic atrophy.

Secondary optic atrophy follows prolonged papilloedema, particularly the vintage stage, with continued peripheral constriction of the visual field to involve the central macular fibres, leading to blindness (Fig. 6.25). Figure 6.26 shows progression of visual field loss through the stages of papilloedema.

Toxic neuropathy

Caecocentral scotomas are a feature of toxic, nutritional and genetic inherited optic neuropathies. Bilateral relatively symmetrical caecocentral scotomas with preservation of the peripheral field are the characteristic field defects encountered in nutritional and/or toxic neuropathy.

Trauma

Visual loss following trauma is usually attributable to contusion or laceration of the optic nerves which occurs acutely at the time of impact. The extent of visual field loss is dependent on the degree of involvement of the optic nerves.

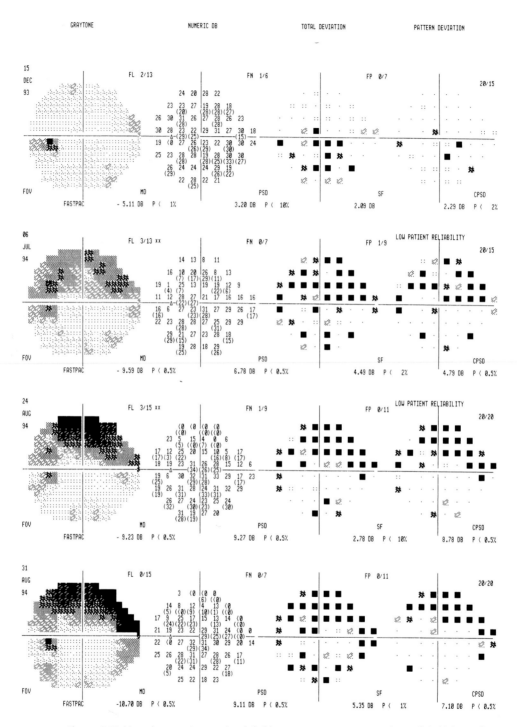

Figure 6.10 Humphrey perimeter visual field assessment: asymmetrical visual field loss (glaucoma). These visual field results show development of a superior arcuate defect and commencement of an inferior arcuate defect in either eye over a period of time.

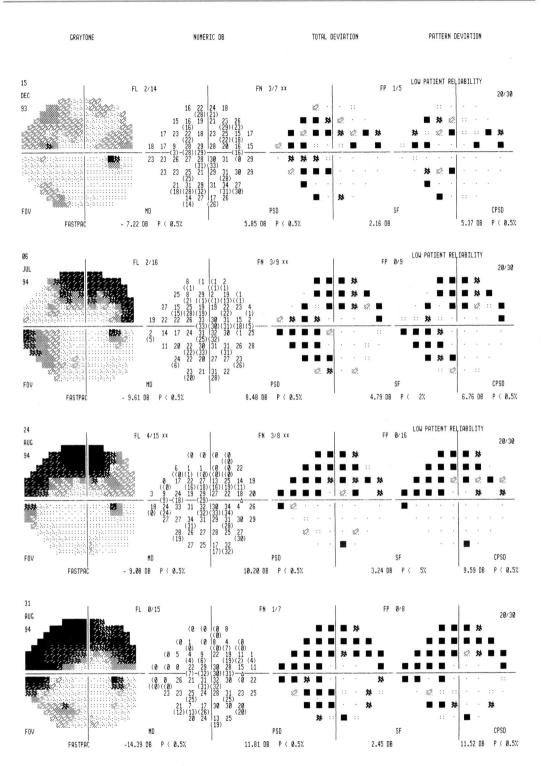

Figure 6.10 (Continued)

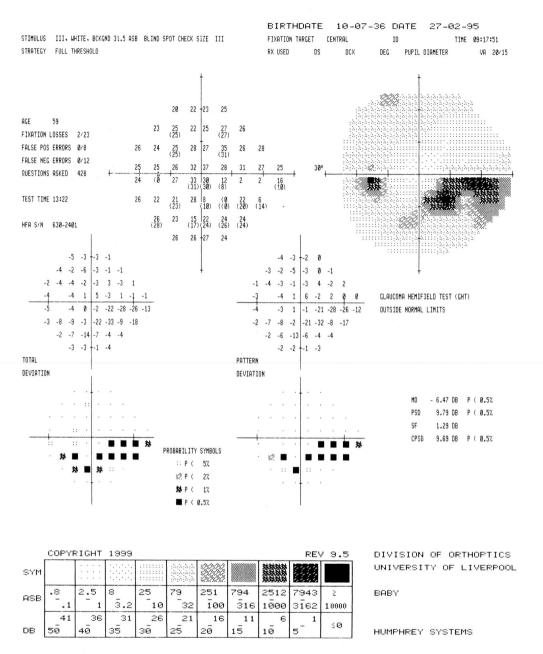

Figure 6.11 Humphrey perimeter visual field assessment: asymmetrical visual field loss (glaucoma). The right eye shows borderline involvement of the inferior visual field near the blind spot. The left eye shows a defined inferior arcuate defect extending to the horizontal meridian with a nasal step.

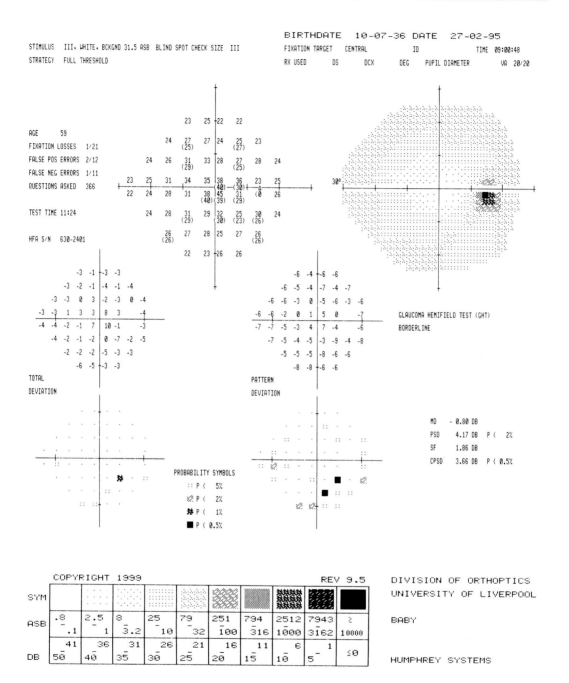

STIMULUS III, WHITE, BCKGND 31.5 ASB BLIND SPOT CHECK SIZE III
STRATEGY FULL THRESHOLD

BIRTHDATE 10-07-36 DATE 27-02-95
FIXATION TARGET CENTRAL ID TIME 09:00:48
RX USED DS DCX DEG PUPIL DIAMETER VA 20/20

AGE 59
FIXATION LOSSES 1/21
FALSE POS ERRORS 2/12
FALSE NEG ERRORS 1/11
QUESTIONS ASKED 366

TEST TIME 11:24

HFA S/N 630-2401

GLAUCOMA HEMIFIELD TEST (GHT)
BORDERLINE

TOTAL
DEVIATION

PATTERN
DEVIATION

MD - 0.80 DB
PSD 4.17 DB P < 2%
SF 1.86 DB
CPSD 3.66 DB P < 0.5%

PROBABILITY SYMBOLS
:: P < 5%
▨ P < 2%
✻ P < 1%
■ P < 0.5%

COPYRIGHT 1999 REV 9.5

SYM		::::	:::::	::::::	:::::	▨▨	▒▒	✻✻	▨▨	■
ASB	.8 – .1	2.5 – 1	8 – 3.2	25 – 10	79 – 32	251 – 100	794 – 316	2512 – 1000	7943 – 3162	≥ 10000
DB	41 50	36 40	31 35	26 30	21 25	16 20	11 15	6 10	1 5	≤0

DIVISION OF ORTHOPTICS
UNIVERSITY OF LIVERPOOL

BABY

HUMPHREY SYSTEMS

Figure 6.11 (Continued)

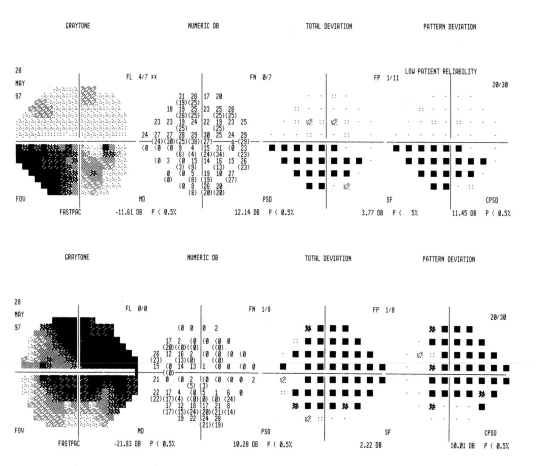

Figure 6.12 Humphrey perimeter visual field assessment: dissimilar patterns of visual field loss (glaucoma). There is a dense inferior arcuate defect in the right eye and dense arcuate defects (superior greater than inferior) in the left eye. Note the decibel values.

THRESHOLD GRAYTONE THRESHOLD (DB) TOTAL DEVIATION PATTERN DEVIATION

20-04-1995 SITA-FAST GHT: OUTSIDE NORMAL LIMITS

```
              29  29  28  28
          30  30  29  29  29  30
      27  30  30  28  28  31  29  27
      28  29  31  31   0   0  29  28  30
      23  17  12  16  (0  (0  27  (0  30
           6  12  15  18  21  28  26  26
               8  12  15  25  29  25
                   7  15  19  11
```

FOVEA: OFF FL: 0/13 FN: 7 % FP: 0 %
MD: -11.48 DB P < 0.5% PSD: 11.30 DB P < 0.5%

10-05-1995 SITA-FAST GHT: WITHIN NORMAL LIMITS

```
              25  30  29  28
          27  29  30  29  29  29
      29  30  32  30  29  30  28  29
      28  28  31  31  33  33  33  30
      26  30  32  33  33  32  29  (0  30
          30  29  32  31  30  31  29  29
              30  31  31  29  31  29
                  31  29  30  29
```

FOVEA: OFF FL: 0/11 FN: 0 % FP: 0 %
MD: -2.23 DB P < 5% PSD: 1.09 DB

THRESHOLD GRAYTONE THRESHOLD (DB) TOTAL DEVIATION PATTERN DEVIATION

20-04-1995 SITA-FAST GHT: WITHIN NORMAL LIMITS

```
              29  29  29  28
          31  29  30  30  30  27
      28  31  32  30  30  31  29  27
      31  22  31  33  33  32  29  29  27
      31  (0  30  32  33  33  31  30  29
          30  30  27  31  32  31  29  29
              29  30  30  31  29  29
                  30  27  30  29
```

FOVEA: OFF FL: 0/10 FN: 0 % FP: 0 %
MD: -2.30 DB P < 5% PSD: 1.22 DB

10-05-1995 SITA-FAST GHT: WITHIN NORMAL LIMITS

```
              30  28  30  30
          30  30  31  32  31  30
      27  29  31  32  33  31  29  29
      30  24  27  32  34  31  31  30  29
      29  (0  30  32  34  33  33  31  28
          27  29  29  31  31  31  28
              29  30  30  31  31  28
                  29  29  27  27
```

FOVEA: OFF FL: 0/11 FN: 0 % FP: 0 %
MD: -2.02 DB P < 5% PSD: 1.43 DB

Figure 6.13 Humphrey perimeter visual field assessment: central scotoma (optic neuritis). There is a right central scotoma with a normal left visual field result. Note 0 decibel values at central fixation. Resolution of visual field loss is the usual outcome – note the improvement within a three week period.

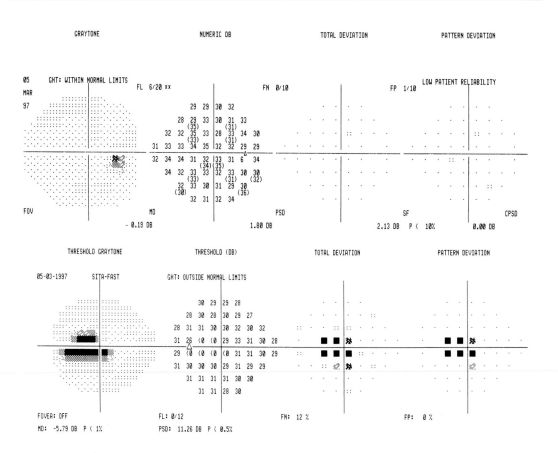

Figure 6.14 Humphrey perimeter visual field assessment: caecocentral scotoma (optic neuritis). There is a left caecocentral central scotoma. Note the reduced decibel values extending from central fixation to the blind spot. The right eye is normal.

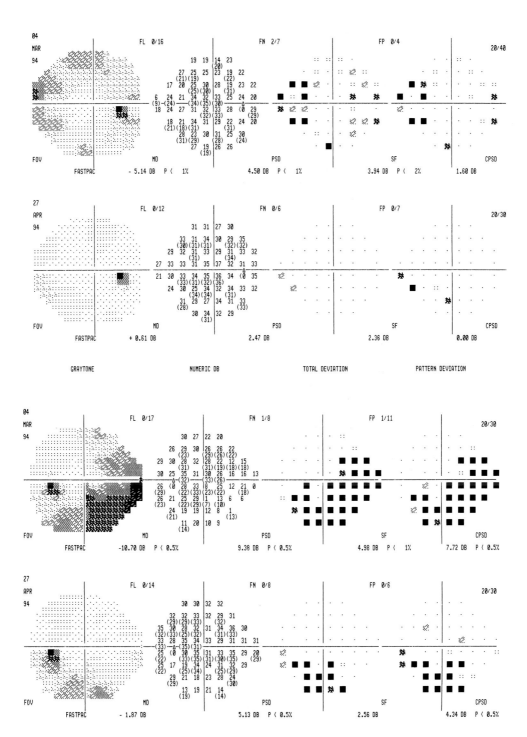

Figure 6.15 Humphrey perimeter visual field assessment: arcuate defect (optic neuritis). There is a mild nasal visual field deficit in the right eye with an inferior arcuate defect and superior nasal visual field deficit in the left eye. There is improvement over a period of time.

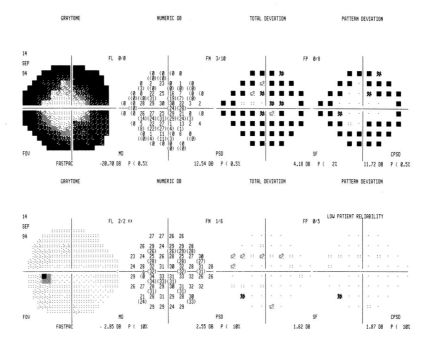

Figure 6.16 Humphrey perimeter visual field assessment: generalised constriction (optic neuritis). There is a constricted right visual field with mild reduced sensitivity only in the left eye.

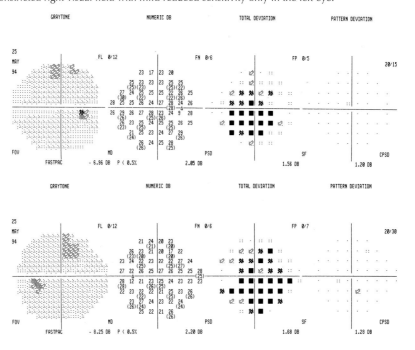

Figure 6.17 Humphrey perimeter visual field assessment: reduced sensitivity (optic neuritis). Bilateral reduced sensitivity is evident on the total deviation plots of either eye with no localised visual field impairment evident on the corrected pattern standard deviation plots.

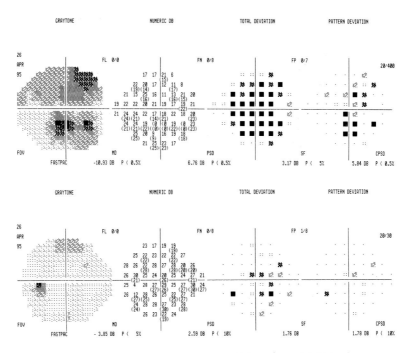

Figure 6.18 Humphrey perimeter visual field assessment: bilateral visual field loss (optic neuritis). The right eye shows reduced sensitivity across the visual field, particularly the inferior paracentral visual field (note the decibel values). The left eye shows reduced sensitivity centrally.

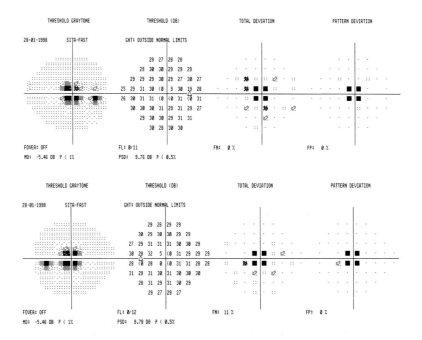

Figure 6.19 Humphrey perimeter visual field assessment: bilateral visual field loss (optic neuritis). There is a central scotoma in either eye. Note the 0 decibel values at central fixation.

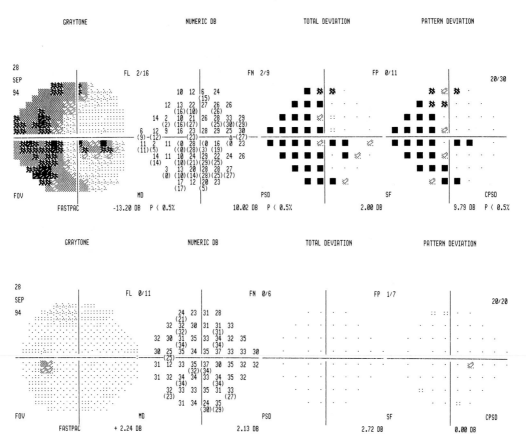

Figure 6.20 Humphrey perimeter visual field assessment: atypical visual field loss (optic neuritis). Right scotomatous visual field loss is present centrally (note the decibel values) along with superior and inferior nasal visual field loss. The left eye result is normal.

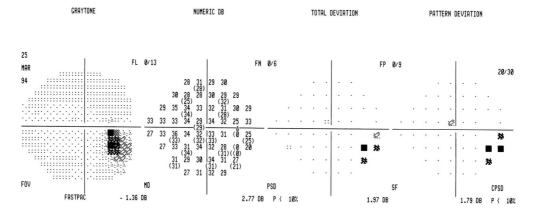

Figure 6.21 Humphrey perimeter visual field assessment: early papilloedema. This patient with idiopathic intracranial hypertension has an enlarged blind spot in the right visual field. Note the extension of the blind spot area with reduced decibel values and probability plots.

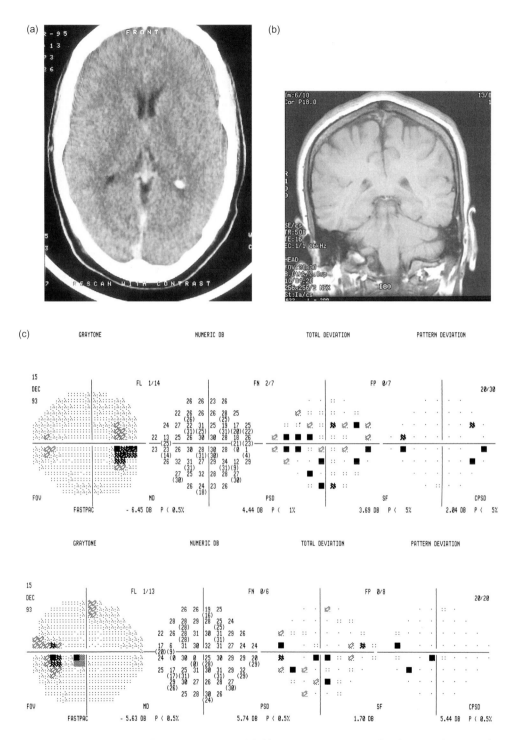

Figure 6.22 Humphrey perimeter visual field assessment: acute papilloedema. In this case of sagittal sinus thrombosis, on neuroimaging (a,b) note the increased signal in the superior sagittal sinus indicating the presence of thrombosis. There is a secondary increase in intracranial pressure as cerebrospinal fluid drainage into the superior sagittal sinus is impaired; papilloedema results. On visual field assessment (c) enlarged blind spots are documented in relation to the papilloedema with some generalised and scotomatous visual field loss predominantly relating to involvement of the nerve fibre layers at the optic disc.

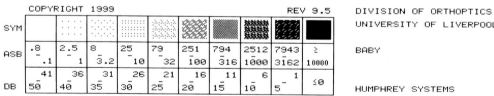

DIVISION OF ORTHOPTICS
UNIVERSITY OF LIVERPOOL

BABY

HUMPHREY SYSTEMS

STIMULUS   III, WHITE, BCKGND 31.5 ASB BLIND SPOT CHECK SIZE III
STRATEGY   FULL THRESHOLD
FASTPAC
LOW PATIENT RELIABILITY

BIRTHDATE   18-02-73 DATE   03-03-94
FIXATION TARGET   CENTRAL   ID 990641   TIME 16:00:48
RX USED   DS   DCX   DEG   PUPIL DIAMETER   VA 20/80

AGE   21
FIXATION LOSSES   0/16
FALSE POS ERRORS   0/7
FALSE NEG ERRORS   5/9 xx
QUESTIONS ASKED   316

TEST TIME 10:20

HFA S/N

TOTAL
DEVIATION

PATTERN
DEVIATION

MD   -23.97 DB   P < 0.5%
PSD   11.59 DB   P < 0.5%
SF   3.76 DB   P < 5%
CPSD   10.87 DB   P < 0.5%

PROBABILITY SYMBOLS
:: P < 5%
⊠ P < 2%
⋇ P < 1%
■ P < 0.5%

COPYRIGHT 1999   REV 9.5

Figure 6.23 Humphrey perimeter visual field assessment: chronic papilloedema. In this case of idiopathic intracranial hypertension, the right eye shows arcuate defects (superior greater than inferior) with relative sparing of the central 10 degrees of visual field (note the decibel values). The left eye shows more marked involvement with constriction of the visual field but relative sparing of the central 5 degrees of the visual field.

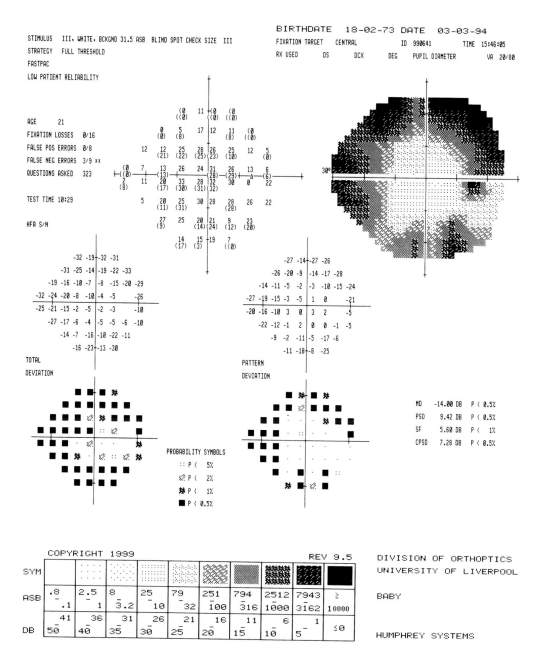

STIMULUS   III, WHITE, BCKGND 31.5 ASB BLIND SPOT CHECK SIZE III
STRATEGY   FULL THRESHOLD
FASTPAC
LOW PATIENT RELIABILITY

BIRTHDATE   18-02-73 DATE   03-03-94
FIXATION TARGET   CENTRAL   ID 990641   TIME 15:46:05
RX USED   DS   DCX   DEG   PUPIL DIAMETER   VA 20/80

AGE   21
FIXATION LOSSES   0/16
FALSE POS ERRORS   0/8
FALSE NEG ERRORS   3/9 xx
QUESTIONS ASKED   323

TEST TIME 10:29

HFA S/N

TOTAL
DEVIATION

PATTERN
DEVIATION

PROBABILITY SYMBOLS

:: P < 5%
▨ P < 2%
✴ P < 1%
■ P < 0.5%

MD   -14.00 DB   P < 0.5%
PSD   9.42 DB   P < 0.5%
SF   5.60 DB   P < 1%
CPSD   7.28 DB   P < 0.5%

COPYRIGHT 1999   REV 9.5

DIVISION OF ORTHOPTICS
UNIVERSITY OF LIVERPOOL

BABY

HUMPHREY SYSTEMS

SYM										
ASB	.8 - .1	2.5 - 1	8 - 3.2	25 - 10	79 - 32	251 - 100	794 - 316	2512 - 1000	7943 - 3162	≥ 10000
DB	41 - 50	36 - 40	31 - 35	26 - 30	21 - 25	16 - 20	11 - 15	6 - 10	1 - 5	≤0

Figure 6.23 (Continued)

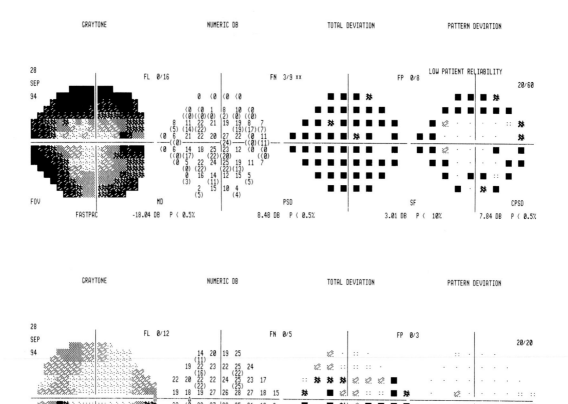

Figure 6.24 Humphrey perimeter visual field assessment: chronic papilloedema. In this case of hydro-cephalus there is asymmetrical visual field impairment. The right visual field is constricted with relative sparing of the central 10 degrees. The left eye shows an enlarged blind spot and an inferior arcuate defect which is more evident on the total probability plot.

Tumours

Visual field defects are due to mechanical compression resulting in nerve fibre bundle defects, generalised depression or scotomas, dependent on the area of nerve compressed. The defects are variable and may include nerve fibre destruction and vascular compromise. Generally, the central visual field will be involved; visual field loss is often unilateral (Fig. 6.27) but may also occur bilaterally (Fig. 6.2b).

Apart from compression of the optic nerve caused by tumours, compression may also result from paranasal sinus masses which involve the optic canals as the mass enlarges, or from inflammation of the optic nerve. Visual field defects take the form of central scotomas, with or without peripheral constriction of the visual field.

Compression of the optic nerve may also occur with a crowded orbital apex in thyroid eye disease (Fig. 6.1). Visual fields demonstrate central scotomas which are often combined with nerve fibre bundle defects (Figs 6.28 and 6.29). The visual field loss is often bilateral due to bilateral disease, but can be quite asymmetrical in its extent. With prompt diagnosis and immediate intervention, the outcome can be very satisfactory with resolution of much of the visual field loss.

Vascular abnormalities

Ischaemic optic neuropathy with infarction of the disc is a common cause of sudden loss of vision, especially in the older population. Visual field defects vary, but usually take the form of arcuate scotomas or altitudinal hemianopias (Fig. 6.30) of the superior or inferior half of the visual fields. The altitudinal defects are dense and easily discovered. Central scotomas are the predominant field defects in a number of cases, but are often combined with nerve fibre bundle defects (Fig. 6.31). It is not uncommon for optic atrophy to develop as optic disc oedema resolves (Colour Plate 6.14). The visual field loss does not tend to recover.

Choice of visual field assessment

Central visual field assessment is usually sufficient to detect most field defects in optic nerve disease, particularly in glaucoma. If glaucoma is suspected but there

(a)

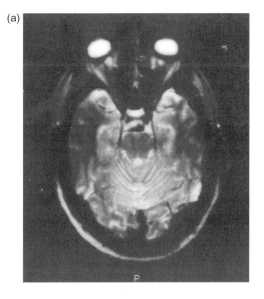

Figure 6.25 Humphrey perimeter visual field assessment: optic atrophy. (a) On neuroimaging of this case of idiopathic intracranial hypertension, enlarged optic nerves consistent with accumulation of cerebrospinal fluid around each nerve can be seen. (b) Visual field assessment reveals there is bilateral constriction of the visual field with reduction of the central 5 degrees of visual field also. Note the reduced decibel values (right greater than left).

(b)

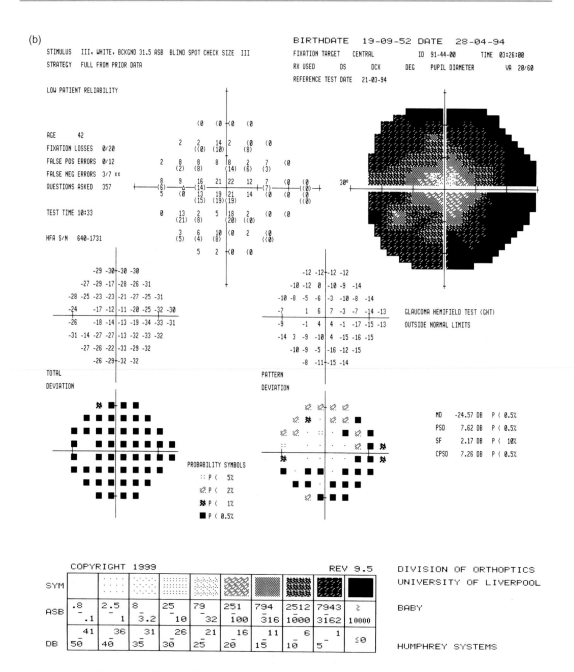

Figure 6.25 (Continued)

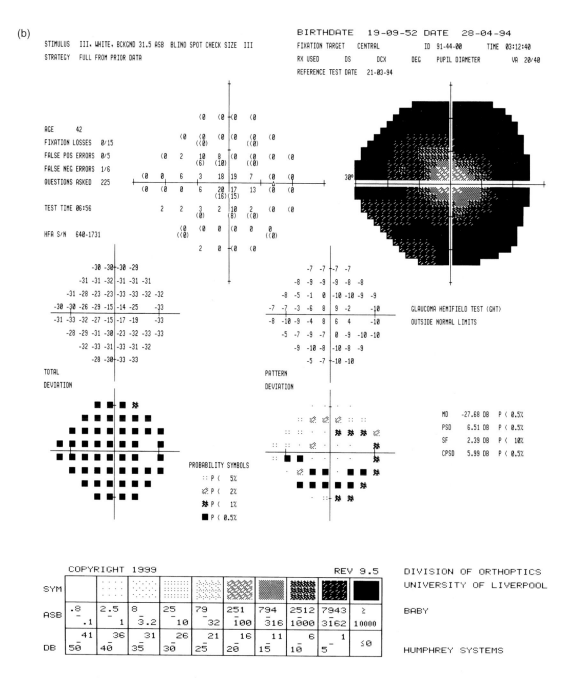

Figure 6.25 (Continued)

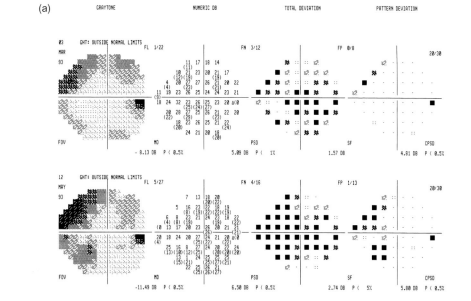
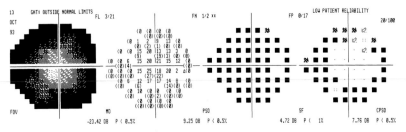
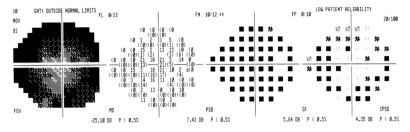
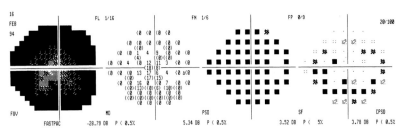

Figure 6.26 Humphrey perimeter visual field assessment: progressive papilloedema. This case of idiopathic intracranial hypertension shows relatively rapid progression of visual field loss over a one year period (a). The right eye shows early reduced sensitivity, particularly in the nasal visual field, with development of arcuate defects (superior greater than inferior) and eventually constriction of the visual field where the central area remains initially spared but is also then involved over time. The change analysis (b) shows deepening of the boxplot, a fall in the mean deviation slope, and initial decrease and then increase of the pattern standard deviation and corrected pattern standard deviation graphs as the hill of vision changes from localised to generalised loss of sensitivity.

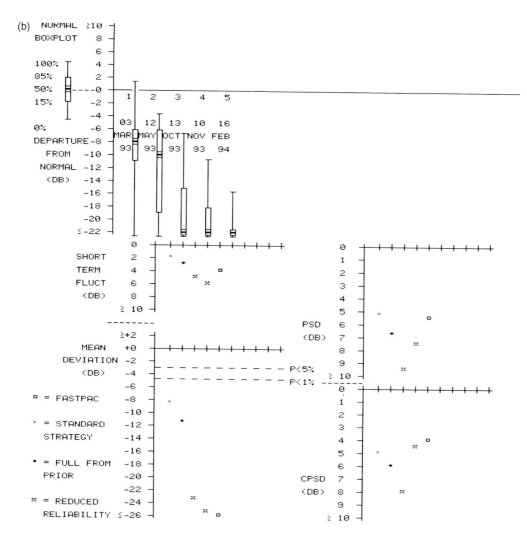

Figure 6.26 (Continued)

are no visual field defects centrally, a peripheral visual field test may demonstrate a nasal step. Where the visual field is constricted in late disease, a central 10 degree programme should be chosen to document any remaining visual field.

Where there is suspected temporal visual field loss, it is advisable to choose a peripheral visual field assessment to explore this area, e.g. in cases of temporal wedge sector loss with optic nerve hypoplasia.

In the diagnostic stages of optic nerve disease follow-up may be required every 3 months. Follow-up for patients with change in their visual status is generally 3–6 monthly. Stable visual status requires follow-up at 6–12 monthly intervals. Long-term stability typically requires yearly follow-up.

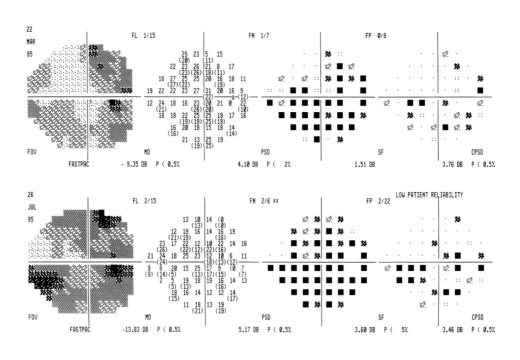

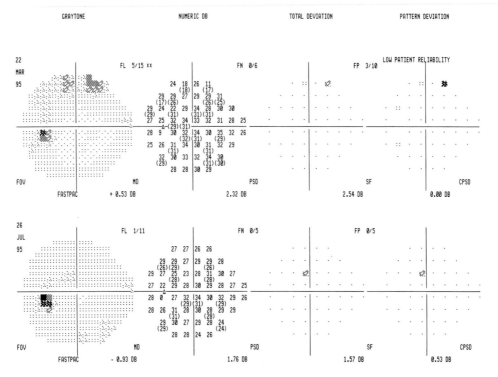

Figure 6.27 Humphrey perimeter visual field assessment: unilateral optic nerve meningioma. The right eye shows progressive visual field loss with temporal and inferior nasal involvement initially, developing to generalised constriction. The left eye result is normal.

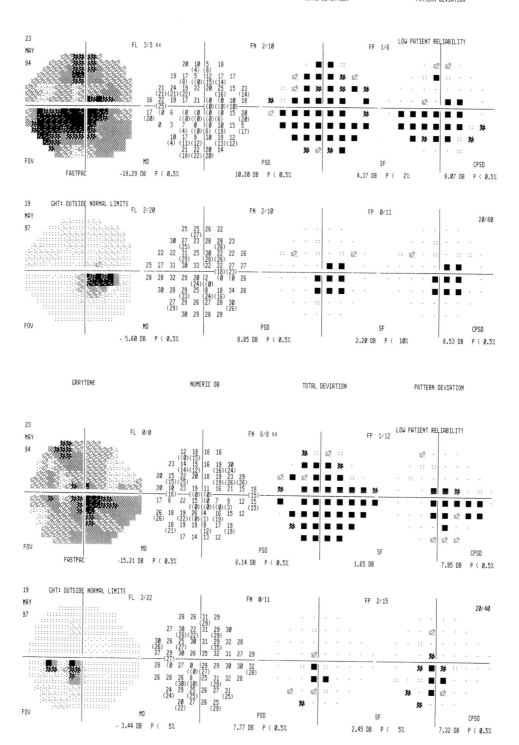

Figure 6.28 Humphrey perimeter visual field assessment: thyroid eye disease. In either eye there is a central scotoma but with involvement of the nasal inferior visual field also. This is seen to improve slowly over time following medical treatment, leaving residual bilateral central scotomas.

GRAYTONE   NUMERIC DB   TOTAL DEVIATION   PATTERN DEVIATION

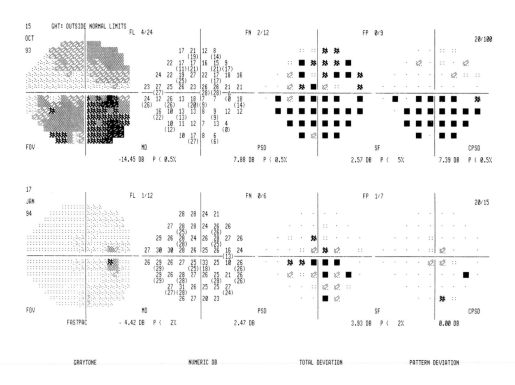

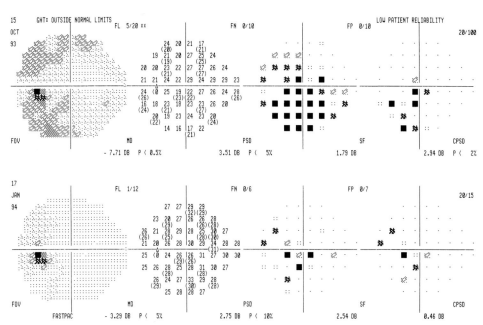

Figure 6.29 Humphrey perimeter visual field assessment: thyroid eye disease. There is bilateral reduced sensitivity, particularly the inferior visual field (right greater than left). Note the decibel values and probability plots. There is improvement of visual field function over follow-up, with residual reduced sensitivity of the central visual field only.

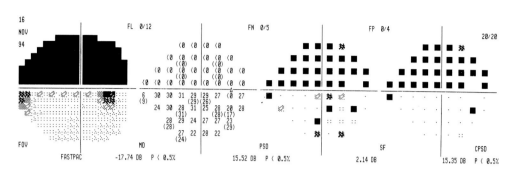

Figure 6.30 Humphrey perimeter visual field assessment: altitudinal defect (vascular). There is a right altitudinal visual field defect which respects the horizontal meridian, with involvement of both nasal and temporal superior visual field quadrants. Note the sensitivity values of 0 decibels above the horizontal meridian. This visual field defect is due to a vascular abnormality with infarction of the inferior branch of the central retinal artery.

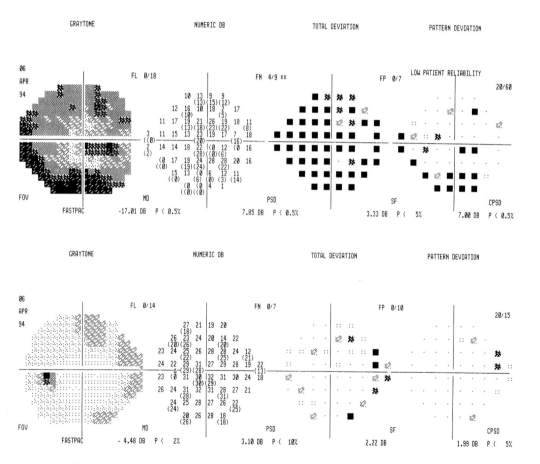

Figure 6.31 Humphrey perimeter visual field assessment: nerve fibre bundle defects (vascular). In this case of anterior ischaemic optic neuropathy, note the involvement of the right eye with constriction of the visual field, but in particular the nasal field of vision. There is a central scotoma (note 0 decibel values). The left eye shows some spurious mild nasal visual field involvement.

References

Anderson DR (1970) Ultrastructure of the optic nerve head. *Archives of Ophthalmology*, **83**: 63

Asman P, Heijl A (1992) Glaucoma hemifield test. Automated visual field evaluation. *Archives of Ophthalmology*, **110**: 812

Brazitikos PD, Safran AB, Simona F, Zulauf M (1990) Threshold perimetry in tilted disc syndrome. *Archives of Ophthalmology*, **108**: 1698

Brown GC, Shields JA, Goldberg RE (1980) Congenital pits of the optic nerve head. II. Clinical studies in humans. *Ophthalmology*, **87**: 51

Buchanan TA, Hoyt WF (1981) Temporal visual field defects associated with nasal hypoplasia of the optic disc. *British Journal of Ophthalmology*, **65**: 636

Chou PI, Sadun AA, Lee H (1995) Vasculature and morphometry of the optic canal and intracanalicular optic nerve. *Journal of NeuroOphthalmology*, **15**: 186

Cioffi GA, van Buskirk EM. (1994) Microvasculature of the anterior optic nerve. *Survey of Ophthalmology*, **38**: 107

Drance SM (1972) The glaucomatous visual field. *British Journal of Ophthalmology*, **56**: 186

Eustis HS, Sanders MR, Zimmermann T (1994) Morning glory syndrome in children. *Archives of Ophthalmology*, **112**: 204

Flanagan P, Zele AJ (2004) Chromatic and luminance losses with multiple sclerosis and optic neuritis measured using dynamic random luminance contrast noise. *Ophthalmic and Physiological Optics*, **24**: 225

Foulds WS, Chisholm IA, Bronte-Stewart J, Reid HCR (1970) Investigation and therapy of the toxic amblyopics. *Transactions of the Ophthalmic Societies of the UK*, **90**: 739

Francois J, Neetens A (1954) Vascularisation of optic pathway I. Lamina cribrosa and optic nerve. *British Journal of Ophthalmology*, **38**: 472

Francois J, Neetens A (1963) Central retinal artery and central optic nerve artery. *British Journal of Ophthalmology*, **47**: 21

Francois J, Neetans A, Collette JM (1955) Vascular supply of the optic pathway II. Further studies by micro-arteriography of the optic nerve. *British Journal of Ophthalmology*, **39**: 220

Gasser P, Flammer J (1986) Optic neuropathy of Grave's disease: a report of a perimetric follow-up. *Ophthalmologica*, **192**: 22

Guiffre G (1986) The spectrum of the visual field defects in the tilted disc syndrome: clinical study and review. *Neuroophthalmology*, **6**: 239

Gutteridge IF, Cockburn DM (1981) Optic nerve head drusen: a correlation of clinical signs. *Australian Journal of Optometry*, **64**: 252

Hart WM, Becker B (1982) The onset and evolution of glaucomatous visual field defects. *Ophthalmology*, **89**: 268

Hayreh SS, Revie HIS, Edwards J (1970) Vasogenic origin of visual field defects and optic nerve changes in glaucoma. *British Journal of Ophthalmology*, **54**: 461

Heijl A, Patella VM (2002) *The Field Analyzer Primer. Essential Perimetry*, 3rd edn. Dublin, CA, Carl Zeiss Meditec

Katz J, Quigley HA, Sommer A (1996) Detection of incident field loss using the glaucoma hemifield test. *Ophthalmology*, **103**: 657

Kerrigan-Baumrind LA, Quigley HA, Pease ME, Kerrigan DF, Mitchell RS (2000) Number of ganglion cells in glaucoma eyes compared with threshold visual field tests in the same persons. *Investigative Ophthalmology and Visual Science*, **41**: 741

Lambert SR, Hoyt CS, Narahara MH (1987) Optic nerve hypoplasia. *Survey of Ophthalmology*, **32**: 1

Pollock S (1987) The morning glory disc anomaly: contractile movement, classification and embryogenesis. *Documenta Ophthalmologica*, **65**: 439

Radius RL, Anderson DL (1979a) The histology of retinal nerve fibre layer bundles and bundle defects. *Archives of Ophthalmology*, **97**: 948

Radius RL, Anderson DL (1979b) The course of axons through the retina and optic nerve head. *Archives of Ophthalmology*, **97**: 1154

Roh S, Noecker RJ, Schuman JS, Hedges TR, Weiter JJ, Mattox C (1998) Effect of optic nerve head drusen on nerve fibre layer thickness. *Ophthalmology*, **105**: 878

Sadun A, Currie JN, Lessell S (1984) Transient visual obscurations with elevated optic discs. *Annals of Neurology*, **16**: 489

Schneck ME, Haegerstrom-Portnoy G (1997) Color vision defect type and spatial vision in the optic neuritis treatment trial. *Investigative Ophthalmology and Visual Science*, **38**: 2278

Stewart WC, Shields MB (1991) The peripheral visual field in glaucoma: re-evaluation in the age of automated perimetry. *Survey of Ophthalmology*, **36**: 59

Tso MOM (1981) Pathology and pathogenesis of drusen of the optic nerve head. *Ophthalmology*, **88**: 1066

Further reading

Adler H, Kaufman PL (eds) (2002) *Adler's Physiology of the Eye. Clinical Application*, 10th edn. St Louis, Mosby

Airaksinen PJ, Drance SM, Douglas GR, Schulzer M, Wijsman K (1985) Visual field and retinal nerve fibre layer comparisons in glaucoma. *Archives of Ophthalmology*, **103**: 205

Anderson DR (1983) What happens to the optic disc and retina in glaucoma? *Ophthalmology*, **90**: 766

Apple DJ, Rabb MF, Walsh PM (1982) Congenital anomalies of the optic disc. *Survey of Ophthalmology*, **27**: 3

Armaly MF (1969) Ocular pressure and visual fields. *Archives of Ophthalmology*, **81**: 25

Balazsi AG, Rootman J, Drance SM, Schulzer M, Douglas GR (1984) The effect of age on the nerve fibre population of the human optic nerve. *American Journal of Ophthalmology*, **97**: 760

Bayer A, Erb C (2002) Short-wavelength automated perimetry, frequency-doubling technology perimetry and pattern-ERG for prediction of progressive glaucomatous standard visual field defects. *Ophthalmology*, **109**: 1009

Beri M, Klugman MR, Kohler JA, Hayreh SS (1975) Anterior ischaemic optic neuropathy. VII. Incidence of bilaterality and various influencing factors. *Ophthalmology*, **94**: 1020

Boghen DR, Glaser JS (1975) Ischemic optic neuropathy. *Brain*, **98**: 699

Boone MI, Massry GG, Frankel RA, Holds JB, Chung SM (1996) Visual outcome in bilateral nonarteritic anterior ischaemic optic neuropathy. *Ophthalmology*, **103**: 1223

Brodsky MC (1994) Congenital optic disk anomalies. *Survey of Ophthalmology*, **39**: 89

Brown GC, Shields JA (1985) Tumors of the optic nerve head. *Survey of Ophthalmology*, **29**: 239

Brouwer B, Zeeman WPC (1925) Experimental anatomical investigation concerning the projection of the retina on the primary optic centres in apes. *Journal of Neurology and Pscychiatry*, **6**: 1

Brouwer B, Zeeman WPC (1926) The projection of the retina in the primary optic neuron in monkeys. *Brain*, **49**: 1

Caprioli J, Sears M, Spaeth GL (1986) Comparison of visual field defects in normal-tension glaucoma and high-tension glaucoma. *American Journal of Ophthalmology*, **102**: 402

Cashwell LF, Ford JG (1995) Central visual field changes associated with acquired pits of the optic nerve. *Ophthalmology*, **102**: 1270

Chamlin M (1953) Visual changes in optic neuritis. *Archives of Ophthalmology*, **50**: 699

Cleary PA, Beck RW, Bourque LB, Backlund JC, Miskala PH (1997) Visual symptoms after optic neuritis: results from the optic neuritis treatment trial. *Journal of NeuroOphthalmology*, **17**: 18

Corbett JJ, Savino PJ, Thompson HS, Kansu T, Schatz NJ, Orr LS, Hopson D (1982) Visual loss in pseudotumor cerebri: follow-up of 57 patients from five to 41 years and a profile of 14 patients with permanent severe visual loss. *Archives of Neurology*, **39**: 461

Cox TA, Haskins GE, Gangitano JL, Antonson DL (1983) Bilateral Toxocara optic neuropathy. *Journal of Clinical NeuroOphthalmology*, **3**: 267

Donovan A (1967) The nerve fibre composition of the cat optic nerves. *Journal of Anatomy*, **101**: 1

Drance SM, Douglas GR, Airaksinen PJ, Schulzer M, Hitchings RA (1987) Diffuse visual field loss in chronic open-angle and low-tension glaucoma. *American Journal of Ophthalmology*, **104**: 577

Dutton JJ (1992) Optic nerve sheath meningiomas. *Survey of Ophthalmology*, **37**: 167

Dutton JJ (1994) Gliomas of the anterior visual pathway. *Survey of Ophthalmology*, **38**: 427

Ernest JT (1975) Pathogenesis of glaucomatous optic nerve disease. *Transactions of American Ophthalmic Society*, **73**: 366

Fish RH, Hoskins JC, Kline LB (1993) Toxoplasmosis neuroretinitis. *Ophthalmology*, **100**: 1177

Flammer J, Drance JM, Augustiny L, Funkhouser A (1985) Quantification of glaucomatous visual field defects with automated perimetry. *Investigative Ophthalmology and Visual Science*, **26**: 176

Frisen L, Royt WF, Tengroth BM (1973) Optociliary veins, disc pallor and visual loss. *Acta Ophthalmologica*, **51**: 241

Glaser JS (1967) The nasal visual field. *Archives of Ophthalmology*, **77**: 358

Gopal L, Badrinath SS, Kumar KS, Doshi G, Biswas N (1996) Optic disc in fundus coloboma. *Ophthalmology*, **103**: 2120

Grimson BS, Perry DD (1984) Enlargement of the optic disc in childhood optic nerve tumors. *American Journal of Ophthalmology*, **97**: 627

Hayreh SS (1974) Anatomy and physiology of the optic nerve head. *Transactions of American Academy of Ophthalmology and Otolaryngology*, **78**: 240

Hayreh SS, Podhajsky PZ, Zimmerman B (1997) Nonarteritic anterior ischaemic optic neuropathy: time of onset of visual loss. *American Journal of Ophthalmology*, **124**: 641

Hayreh SS, Podhajsky P (1979) Visual field defects in anterior ischaemic optic neuropathy. *Documenta Ophthalmigica Proceedings Series*, **19**: 53

Hedges TR, Legge RH, Peli E, Yardley CJ (1995) Retinal nerve fiber layer loss in idiopathic intracranial hypertension. *Ophthalmology*, **102**: 1242

Henson DB, Chaudry S, Artes PH, Faragher EB, Ansons A (2000) Response variability in the visual field: comparison of optic neuritis, glaucoma, ocular hypertension and normal eyes. *Investigative Ophthalmology and Visual Science*, **41**: 417

Hoyt WF, Beeston D (1966) *The Ocular Fundus in Neurologic Disease*. St Louis, Mosby

Hoyt WF, Luis O (1962) Visual fiber anatomy in the infrageniculate pathway of the primate: uncrossed and crossed retinal quadrant fiber projections studies with Nauta silver stain. *Archives of Ophthalmology*, **68**: 94

Hoyt WF, Tudor RC (1963) The course of papillary temporal retinal axons through the anterior optic nerve. A Nanta degeneration study in the primate. *Archives of Ophthalmology*, **69**: 503

Hughes B (1958) Blood supply of the optic nerve and chiasm and its clinical significance. *British Journal of Ophthalmology*, **42**: 106

Hughes D (1954) *The Visual Fields: A Study of the Applications of Quantitative Perimetry to the Anatomy and Pathology of the Visual Pathways*. Oxford, Blackwell Science

Jacobson DM, Warner JJ, Broste SK (1997) Optic nerve contact and compression by the carotid artery in asymptomatic patients. *American Journal of Ophthalmology*, **123**: 677

Kanski J (2003) *Clinical Ophthalmology. A Systematic Approach*, 5th edn. London, Butterworth Heinemann

Kanski J (2004) *Clinical Ophthalmology. A Synopsis*, London, Butterworth Heinemann/ Elsevier Science

Katz J, Gilbert D, Quigley HA, Sommer A (1996) Estimating progression of visual field loss in glaucoma. *Ophthalmology*, **104**: 1017

Keltner JL, Johnson CA, Spurr JO, Beck RW (1994) Visual field profile of optic neuritis: one year follow-up in the optic neuritis treatment trial. *Archives of Ophthalmology*, **112**: 946

Kline LB (1988) Progression of visual field defects in ischaemic optic neuropathy. *American Journal of Ophthalmology*, **106**: 199

McDonnell P, Miller NR (1983) Chiasmatic and hypothalamic extension of optic nerve glioma. *Archives of Ophthalmology*, **101**: 1412

Mikelberg FS, Drance SM (1984) The mode of progression of visual field defects in glaucoma. *American Journal of Ophthalmology*, **98**: 443

Moody TA, Irvine AR, Cahn PH, Susac JO, Horton JC (1993) Sudden visual field constriction associated with optic disc drusen. *Journal of Clinical NeuroOphthalmology*, **13**: 8

Mustonen E (1983) Pseudopapilloedema with and without verified optic disc drusen: a clinical analysis II. Visual fields. *Acta Ophthalmologica*, **61**: 1057

Neigel JM, Rootman J, Belkin RI, Nugent RA, Drance SM, Beattie CW, Spinelli JA (1988) Dysthyroid optic neuropathy: the crowded orbital apex syndrome. *Ophthalmology*, **95**: 1515

Olver J, Cassidy L (2004) *Ophthalmology at a Glance*. Oxford, Blackwell Publishing

Olver JM, Spalton DJ, McCartney AC (1994) Quantitative morphology of human retro-laminar optic nerve vasculature. *Investigative Ophthalmology and Visual Science*, **35**: 3858

Onda E, Cioffi GA, Bacon DR, Buskirk van EM (1995) Microvasculature of the human optic nerve. *American Journal of Ophthalmology*, **120**: 92

Patterson VH, Heron JR (1980) Visual field abnormalities in multiple sclerosis. *Journal of Neurology, Neurosurgery and Psychiatry*, **43**: 205

Quigley HA, Addicks EM (1982) Quantitative studies of nerve fibre layer defects. *Archives of Ophthalmology*, **100**: 807

Quigley HA, Dunkelberger GR, Green WR (1989) Retinal ganglion cell atrophy correlated with automated perimetry in human eyes with glaucoma. *American Journal of Ophthalmology*, **107**: 453

Salz JJ, Donin JF (1972) Blindness after burns. *Canadian Journal of Ophthalmology*, **7**: 243

Sample PA, Weinreb RN (1990) Color perimetry for assessment of primary open angle glaucoma. *Investigative Ophthalmology and Visual Science*, **31**: 1869

Savino PJ, Glaser JS, Rosenberg MA (1979) A clinical analysis of pseudopapilloedema. II. Visual field defects. *Archives of Ophthalmology*, **97**: 71

Sears ML (1979) Visual field loss in glaucoma. *American Journal of Ophthalmology*, **88**: 493

Seeley R, Smith JL (1972) Visual field defects in optic nerve hypoplasia. *American Journal of Ophthalmology*, **73**: 882

Shaw HE, Smith JL (1980) Cecocentral scotomas – neuro-ophthalmologic considerations. Paper given at *Neuro-ophthalmology Focus*, New York

Shukovsky LJ, Fletcher GH (1973) Retinal and optic nerve complications in a high dose irradiation technique of ethmoid sinus and nasal cavity. *Radiology*, **104**: 629

Snell RS, Lemp MA (1998) *Clinical Anatomy of the Eye*, 2nd edn. Oxford, Blackwell Publishing

Spencer WH (1978) Drusen of the optic disc and aberrant axoplasmic transport. *American Journal of Ophthalmology*, **85**: 1

Steinsapir KD, Goldberg RA (1994) Traumatic optic neuropathy. *Survey of Ophthalmology*, **38**: 487

Stoll MR (1950) Pericentral ring scotoma. *Archives of Ophthalmology*, **43**: 66

Takashima M, Kani K (1995) Receptive fields of retinal ganglion cells and visual fields. In: *Transactions of 8th International Orthoptic Congress*, p. 363

Traquair HM (1949) *An Introduction to Clinical Perimetry*. London, Kimpton

Van Crevel H, Verhaart WJC (1963) The rate of secondary degeneration in the central nervous system. II. The optic nerve of the cat. *Journal of Anatomy*, **97**: 451

Wall M, George D (1987) Visual loss in pseudotumor cerebri: incidence and defects related to visual field strategy. *Archives of Neurology*, **44**: 170

Chapter 7

Optic chiasm

Anatomy*

The optic chiasm is approximately 13 mm wide and is formed by the mergence of the two optic nerves. It is attached by the pia mater and the arachnoid to the dorsal surface of the diencephalon and it forms a portion of the floor of the third ventricle. Its posterior surface is in close contact with the tuber cinereum, it is superior to the tuberculum sellae turcicae and the diaphragma sellae and is usually posterior to the optic groove of the sphenoid bone (Fig. 7.1). It is closely related to the internal carotid arteries and anterior communicating artery anteriorly.

Crossed and uncrossed retinal nerve fibres begin to separate at the termination of the optic nerve at the anterior angle of the optic chiasm. Wilbrand (1929) claimed that the crossed fibres, from nasal retina, lie medial to the pial septum. The inferior crossed fibres, primarily peripheral, remain inferior; after decussating, they loop anteriorly into the terminal portion of the opposite optic nerve (Wilbrand's knee) before turning posteriorly to continue through the optic chiasm and into the optic tract. Doubt has been cast as to the presence of Wilbrand's knee following anatomical studies (Horton 1997). Superior crossing fibres pass posteriorly and enter the superomedial ipsilateral optic tract before looping forward to decussate and enter the contralateral optic tract. Uncrossed temporal retinal fibres maintain their relative position at the lateral aspects of the optic chiasm. Nasal macular fibres cross primarily in the central and posterior portions of the optic chiasm.

The blood supply to the optic chiasm is from an anastomosis of arterioles from the Circle of Willis. The dorsal blood supply is mainly from the proximal segments of the anterior cerebral arteries and a lesser supply from the internal carotid and anterior communicating arteries. There are possible contributions from the posterior communicating, posterior cerebral and basilar arteries. Small additional feeders may be supplied by the superior hypoglossal and middle cerebral arteries (Hughes 1958; Bergland & Ray 1969; Wollschlaeger *et al.* 1971).

---

* This anatomy section is intended as a brief description only. If required, further detail should be sought from appropriate textbooks – see Further reading. The anatomy and pathology sections, in combination, provide a background to the part of the visual pathway covered in this chapter so that the relevant visual field defects can be considered and interpreted appropriately.

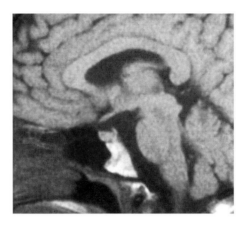

Figure 7.1 Neuroimaging of normal pituitary area. Sagittal view of the middle cranial fossa shows the normal structural layout of the pituitary fossa and optic chiasm situated approximately 1 cm superiorly.

Pathology*

Lesions that compress the optic chiasm include aneurysms, craniopharyngiomas, distension of the third ventricle in obstructive hydrocephalus, optic nerve and chiasmal gliomas and pituitary tumours. Pituitary adenomas are by far the most common pathological lesion involving the optic chiasm.

Resultant visual field defects are due to a combination of direct compression of nerve fibres and interference with the vascular supply to the optic chiasm.

Craniopharyngioma

These are slow growing tumours arising from the vestigal remnants of Rathke's pouch along the pituitary stalk (Fig. 7.2). They occur in all age groups, but particularly children.

Glioma

Gliomas are slow growing tumours typically seen in children, but also presenting in adults and documented frequently with neurofibromatosis (Glaser *et al.* 1971) (Fig. 7.3).

Hydrocephalus

It is important to note that the optic chiasm is situated in the anteroinfero region of the third ventricle. Expanding lesions in this region may compress the hypothalamus

---

* This pathology section is provided as a summary of possible disease processes but by its nature cannot be all inclusive. The reader is directed towards other appropriate textbooks for further detail – see Further reading.

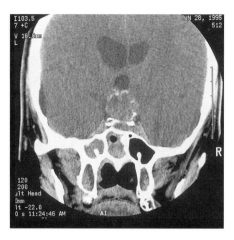

Figure 7.2 Neuroimaging of craniopharyngioma. There is a large central mass above the optic chiasm. This will compress superior retinal fibres first (inferior visual field defect) before involvement of inferior retinal fibres with progressive enlargement of the tumour and further compression of the optic chiasm.

and by distorting the third ventricle and blocking the foramen of Munro, cause elevation of intracranial pressure with subsequent distension and increase in size of the ventricles (Fig. 7.4). Distension of the third ventricle may result in lateral optic chiasm stretching due to lateral splaying of the chiasm against the pulsatile carotid arteries. Enlarged ventricles may also press on the superior aspect of the optic chiasm resulting in inferior visual field defects.

Meningioma

Meningiomas that involve the optic chiasm may arise from the olfactory groove, tuberculum sellae or lesser wing of sphenoid, and are slow growing. These tumours typically affect middle aged women and often cause hyperosmosis which can be seen on a plain skull X-ray. When they arise from the tuberculum sellae, they may compress either the optic nerve or optic chiasm. See Fig. 6.2 for evidence of bilateral visual field loss.

Multiple sclerosis

Demyelination of nerve fibres can occur in the optic chiasm.

Pituitary tumour

Pituitary adenoma is the most common intracranial tumour to involve the optic chiasm. It is a slow growing tumour with insidious visual field loss and endocrine abnormalities as a result of the secreting or non-secreting nature of adenomas

(a)

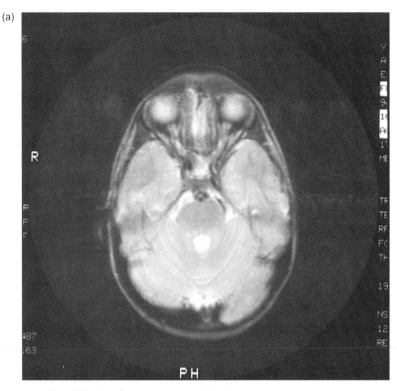

(b)

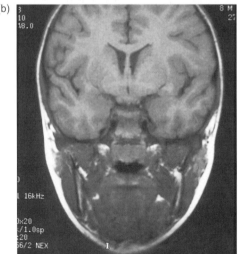

Figure 7.3 Optic chiasm glioma. On neuroimaging note the thickened appearance of the optic chiasm on both (a) transverse and (b) coronal views. On visual field assessment (c) there is predominantly temporal visual field loss in the right eye consistent with optic chiasm involvement and more generalised reduction in visual sensitivity in the left eye.

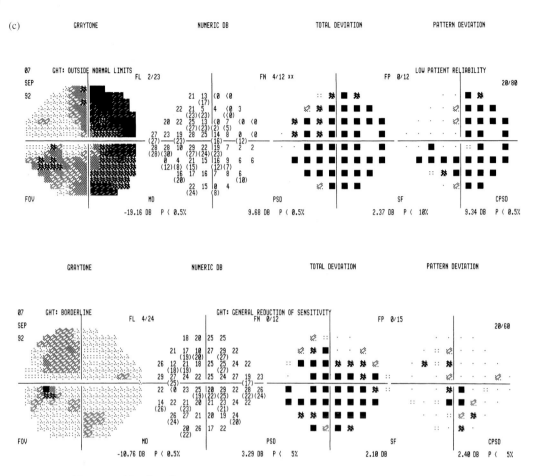

Figure 7.3 (Continued)

(Elkington 1968; Kirkham 1972). The pituitary gland lies in a bony cavity of the sphenoid bone, the sella turcica. The roof of the sella (the diaphragma sellae) is formed by a fold of dura mater which stretches from the anterior clinoids to the posterior clinoids. The optic nerves and the optic chiasm lie above the diaphragma and are therefore susceptible to suprasellar extension of a pituitary tumour (Fig. 7.5). Tumours that remain confined to the sella will not cause visual field defects. Within the optic chiasm, the inferonasal retinal nerve fibres cross low and anteriorly, and therefore are most vulnerable to damage from expanding pituitary lesions. In about 80% of normal subjects, the optic chiasm lies directly above the sella (Bergland *et al.* 1968). In approximately 10% of normal subjects, the optic chiasm is situated more anteriorly, over the tuberculum sellae (prefixed). Another anatomical variation present in the remaining 10% of cases is a postfixed optic chiasm where the chiasm is located more posteriorly over the dorsum sellae. The optic nerves thus have a long intracranial course and as a result pituitary tumours are more likely to present with compression of the optic nerves.

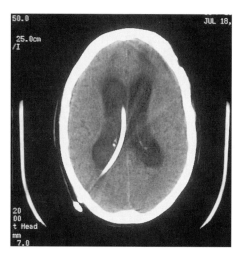

Figure 7.4 Neuroimaging of hydrocephalus. Typical enlarged lateral ventricles are evident. The white tube is a ventriculoperitoneal shunt.

(a)

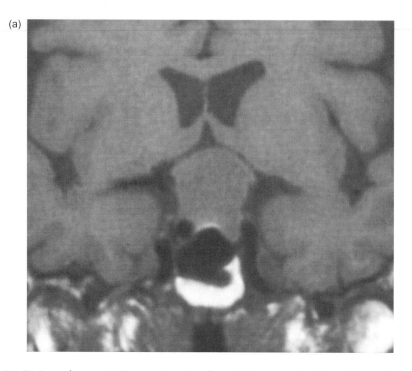

Figure 7.5 Pituitary adenoma. (a) On neuroimaging a large pituitary mass is evident with superior extension. The optic chiasm is stretched and splayed across the superior aspect of the tumour extension. (b) On visual field assessment there is bilateral temporal visual field loss (superior greater than inferior as the tumour compresses inferior retinal nerve fibres first). Note the decibel values and probability plots. Either eye respects the vertical meridia.

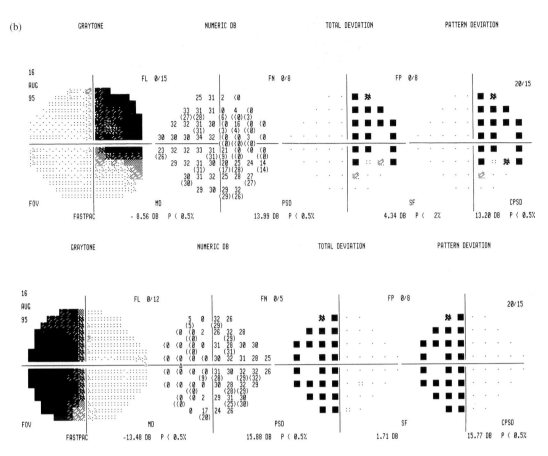

Figure 7.5 (Continued)

Rapid expansion of the tumour because of haemorrhage from it or within it results in pituitary apoplexy .

Trauma

Optic chiasm damage secondary to trauma is rare and usually surgically induced. It can also be due to direct severe frontal head trauma.

Vascular abnormalities

Aneurysms arising from the intracavernous portion of the internal carotid artery may erode into the sella and mimic pituitary tumours (Fig. 7.6). For this reason, it is wise to perform carotid angiography before surgical exploration of the sella region. As the internal carotid artery curves posteriorly and upwards into the cavernous sinus, it lies immediately below the optic nerves. It then ascends vertically alongside the lateral aspect of the optic chiasm. The precommunicating portion of the anterior cerebral artery is closely related to the anterior surface of the optic chiasm and optic nerves. An aneurysm in this region can therefore compress both the optic nerve and the optic chiasm. A dilatation of an internal carotid aneurysm may cause lateral compression of the optic chiasm. The nasal visual field defect is initially unilateral, but it may become bilateral if the optic chiasm is pushed across against the opposite carotid artery.

Associated signs and symptoms*

General signs

Although they do not secrete hormones, craniopharyngiomas may interfere with hypothalamic function; in children they may cause pituitary dwarfism, diabetes insipidus, delayed sexual development and, occasionally, obesity. Presentation in childhood is commonly associated with hydrocephalus.

Pituitary adenomas occur with and without clinically manifest endocrine activity. Pituitary hormones include adrenocorticotrophic hormone (ACTH), thyroid stimulating hormone (TSH), luteinising hormone (LH), follicle stimulating hormone (FSH), somatotropin (STH) and prolactin. Ensuing non-ocular problems include Cushing syndrome, acromegaly, gigantism, infertility, amenorrhoea, and galactorrhoea.

Ocular defects

Associated ocular signs and symptoms include hemifield slide, fixation blindness, extraocular muscle palsies, optic atrophy and pallor.

Ocular motility problems are less frequently associated with optic chiasm lesions than visual field defects. However, patients may experience symptoms due to a number of ocular motility defects.

Cranial nerve palsy/ocular deviation

Cranial nerve palsies may be seen in association with optic chiasm compression where there is involvement of the cavernous sinus by lateral extension of a pituitary tumour (Chamlin *et al.* 1955) or with an aneurysm. The third, fourth or sixth cranial nerves, or a combination, may be affected, with resulting extraocular muscle involvement and appreciation of diplopia. Secondary strabismus, usually

* This section on associated signs and symptoms is provided so that the practitioner is aware of additional information that can be considered in conjunction with the visual field defect to aid differential diagnosis and localisation of pathology.

exotropia, due to loss of central visual acuity from optic pathway compression has been reported (Chamlin *et al.* 1955; Rowe 1996).

Hemifield slide phenomenon

The hemifield slide phenomenon may account for the appreciation of vertical or horizontal diplopia in the absence of a demonstrable cranial nerve paresis

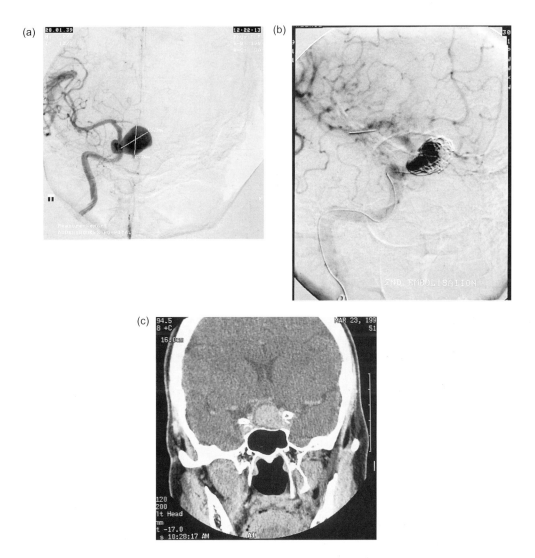

Figure 7.6 Internal carotid artery aneurysm. On neuroimaging the aneurysm is seen clearly on magnetic resonance angiography: (a) preembolisation view; (b) post embolisation view. (c) There is a central mass effect evident on magnetic resonance imaging. (d) On visual field assessment there is predominantly superior nasal visual loss in the right eye with more extensive superior visual field loss of the left eye. Recovery of visual function is evident following embolisation of the aneurysm.

(d)

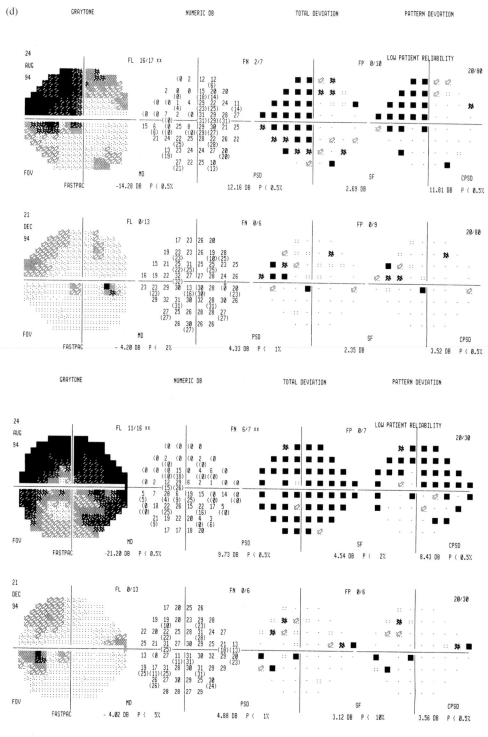

Figure 7.6 (Continued)

(Elkington 1968; Kirkham 1972). Wilson and Falconer (1968) reported that non-paretic diplopia is an early symptom of gross bitemporal hemianopia.

Patients have difficulty in maintaining fusion due to significant reduction in the binocular field (Wybar 1977) and loss of corresponding retinal points (Glaser 1978). The nasal–temporal field overlap of ganglion cell receptive fields ensures a smooth transition of images from nasal to temporal visual field. Patients with bitemporal hemianopia do not have a link between their nasal and temporal visual fields, and where there is a minor extraocular muscle imbalance this may produce vertical or horizontal separation of the two hemifields or overlap of the two hemifields, resulting in intermittent sensory difficulties (Walsh and Hoyt 1982).

Patients with exo deviations have overlap of the visual fields due to crossed projection which occurs on disruption of fusion. Patients with eso deviations have separation of the visual fields and patients with hyper or hypo deviations have vertical separation of images.

Optic atrophy

In addition to assessment of visual fields in patients with optic chiasm lesions, fundus examination is an important part of the ophthalmic investigation. Wilson and Falconer (1968) reported optic atrophy in 56% of their cases. Bow-tie or band atrophy is particularly associated with optic chiasm compression and bitemporal visual field loss. Retinal ganglion axons representing the papillomacular bundle and peripheral nasal retina enter the disc directly. Temporal retinal ganglion axons loop around the papillomacular bundle and enter the disc superiorly and inferiorly. With atrophy of the nasal retinal fibres from an optic chiasm lesion, the retinal nerve fibre layer corresponding to these nasal fibres is lost. The optic disc shows corresponding atrophy at its nasal and temporal aspects, with relative sparing of the superior and inferior aspects where the majority of spared temporal retinal fibres enter.

Post fixational blindness

Post fixational blindness is a condition that occurs with bitemporal hemianopia (Kirkham 1972). When the patient fixates on a near target, there is crossing of the two blind temporal visual fields. This produces a completely blind area of visual field behind the point of fixation. Any object in this area will project to blind nasal retinas and therefore will not be seen by the patient. The patient often has difficulty with visual tasks requiring depth perception (Glaser 1978).

Proptosis

Patients with glioma present with visual field defects and proptosis. Patients with meningioma may have associated cranial nerve palsy or proptosis.

See-saw nystagmus

See-saw nystagmus is a rare condition in which each eye alternately intorts and elevates while the other eye extorts and depresses. Patients appreciate oscillopsia associated with the acquired nystagmus. The association of bitemporal hemianopic visual field defects and see-saw nystagmus probably results from the close proximity of the optic chiasm to the structures involved in producing see-saw nystagmus. Cases of see-saw nystagmus with a bitemporal hemianopia are usually due to tumours of the chiasmal region and suprasellar lesions such as craniopharyngioma.

See-saw nystagmus without bitemporal hemianopia is most probably vascular or congenital in aetiology (Drachman 1966).

Sensory abnormalities

Meningiomas can arise from the sphenoid ridge and compress the optic nerve. Those originating from the olfactory groove may cause a loss of the sense of smell. There may be associated subarachnoid haemorrhage with pituitary apoplexy with severe pain.

Visual acuity

In adults, visual deterioration is the universal symptom with craniopharyngioma. There may be rapid severe unilateral visual loss in adults with glioma. Visual impairment is often the presenting sign of meningioma.

In pituitary apoplexy there are rapidly developing symptoms of sudden profound visual loss.

Asymmetry of visual loss is the rule with pituitary adenoma, to the extent that one eye may show advanced deficits including reduced acuity, whereas only relative temporal field depression is found in the contralateral field. Until acuity is diminished in one or both eyes visual symptoms are absent or vague. The first clue to the presence of a hemianopic defect may be revealed during monocular reading of acuity charts where only half a line of letters is read.

Visual field defects

Most prechiasmal optic neuropathies are due to inflammatory or vascular disease, whereas practically all optic chiasm syndromes are due to pituitary adenomas, other neoplasms or aneurysm compression.

The degree of visual field loss is usually asymmetrical, although the eye with the greater loss usually also has impairment of visual acuity. However, optic atrophy is

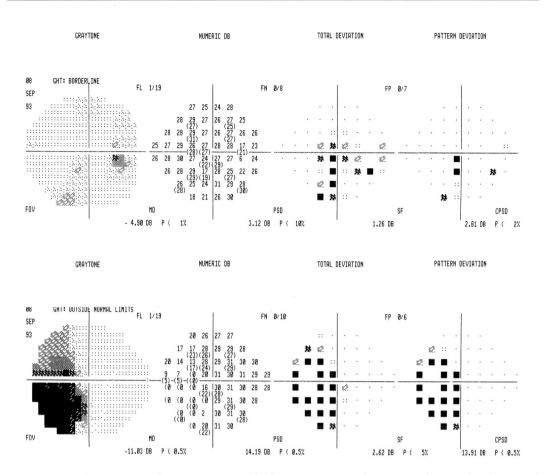

Figure 7.7 Humphrey perimeter visual field assessment: craniopharyngioma. There is right inferior visual field impairment with left temporal visual field impairment (inferior greater than superior as the tumour compresses the superior retinal nerve fibres first). Note the decibel values.

only present in 50% of cases with visual field defects. For this reason, it is extremely important to perform careful examination of the visual fields in all patients with unexplained visual loss.

Compression of the optic chiasm may be symmetrical or asymmetrical relating to the size of lesion and its degree of involvement of the optic chiasm, optic nerve and optic tract. Symmetrical or asymmetrical compression is reflected by the presence of bilateral or unilateral visual field defects.

At the junction of the optic nerve and optic chiasm, the crossed and uncrossed retinal nerve fibres are separated; consequently, a small lesion of the optic nerve at this level affecting either the crossed or the uncrossed fibres may give rise to a unilateral hemianopic defect (Walsh & Gass 1960; Walsh & Hoyt 1982). Hershenfeld and Sharpe (1993) attributed monocular temporal hemifield loss to involvement of the ipsilateral optic nerve close enough to the optic chiasm to impair selectively

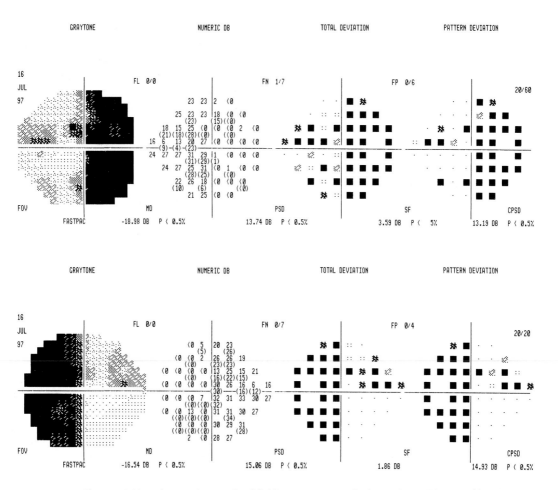

Figure 7.8 Humphrey perimeter visual field assessment: craniopharyngioma. Bitemporal hemianopia is present, with some superior nasal visual field impairment also present bilaterally.

conduction in crossing nasal retinal fibres from the ipsilateral eye, but too anterior to affect the crossing nasal retinal fibres from the contralateral eye.

Sagittal section of the optic chiasm results in bitemporal hemianopia. Direct and consensual pupil reactions remain intact for the nasal visual field. Division of uncrossed retinal nerve fibres leads to binasal hemianopia but represents an unusual lesion (e.g. internal carotid artery aneurysm in the cavernous sinus).

Temporal visual field defects result from compression of the optic chiasm medially involving the crossing of nasal retinal fibres, while nasal visual field defects occur with lateral optic chiasm compression involving the temporal retinal fibres. The visual field defects reported with optic chiasm compression include nasal visual field loss, arcuate visual field defects, scotomatous visual field defects and homonymous visual field loss, in addition to the typical temporal visual field loss (Wilson & Falconer 1968, Rowe *et al.* 1995; Rowe 1998).

Arcuate visual field defects have been proposed to result from vascular changes in the optic nerve rather than at the optic chiasm (Kearns & Rucker 1958). Compression of the optic nerve at the anterior optic chiasm level might also explain the presence of an arcuate defect (Trobe 1974). Trobe (1974) described hemianopic temporal arcuate visual field defects due to a lesion in the anterocentral optic chiasm, where crossing and non-crossing portions of the nerve fibre bundles separate; the lesion would selectively impair crossing fibres. Moller and Hvid-Hansen (1970) supported the concept of mechanical compression of the nerve fibres in the optic nerve and optic chiasm, as opposed to vascular impairment, when explaining the occurrence of visual field defects with optic chiasm lesions. They stated that the nerve fibres in the optic nerve should be regarded as ordinary myelinated fibres, losing their conductability during a variable period if exposed to pressure. Their patients had full recovery of vision and fields which they suggested might not occur if significant loss of vision was caused by vascular obstruction.

Craniopharyngioma

Visual field defects with craniopharyngiomas are frequently asymmetric bitemporal hemianopias or a homonymous pattern with reduced acuity.

Craniopharyngiomas usually compress the optic chiasm superiorly and posteriorly, interfering first with the upper nasal retinal nerve fibres which cross the optic chiasm high and posterior, producing a defect in the inferotemporal quadrants (Fig. 7.7). Scotomatous visual field defects are frequently detected with optic nerve lesions, but may occur with compression of the optic chiasm. The macular nerve fibres decussate throughout the optic chiasm posteriorly and superiorly. For this reason, lesions involving the posterior chiasmal notch, such as craniopharyngiomas, will not only cause inferotemporal field defects but also bitemporal hemianopic scotomas (Wilson & Falconer 1968). With further extension, the visual defect progresses in a clockwise direction in the left eye and anticlockwise in the right eye to involve the upper visual field (Fig. 7.8).

Glioma and meningioma

Meningiomas compressing the junction of the optic chiasm and optic nerve will interfere with the anterior knee of Wilbrand. The crossed and uncrossed retinal fibres are separated at this level within the optic nerve; in addition, there is involvement of the crossed nasal fibres that have briefly looped anteriorly into the involved optic nerve and are situated ventrally, thus being vulnerable to damage from lesions in this area (Wybar 1977; Walsh & Hoyt 1982). A lesion at this site will therefore give rise to an ipsilateral central scotoma and a contralateral upper temporal field defect (junctional scotoma) (Schiefer *et al.* 2004). For this reason, it is very important to test the visual field of the opposite eye in all patients who present with unexplained unilateral visual impairment, particularly including a central visual field defect.

Visual deficits due to meningiomas and gliomas usually take the form of slowly progressive monocular loss of vision. When both fields are involved there is a distinct tendency toward marked asymmetry. Visual field loss typically includes

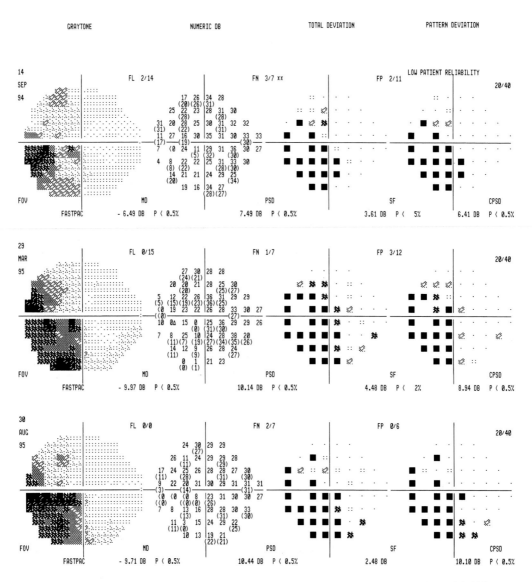

Figure 7.9 Humphrey perimeter visual field assessment: glioma. Progression of visual field loss is seen bilaterally. There is inferior temporal field impairment in either eye – note the decibel values and probability plots. There is an increase in density and progression to involve the superior visual field, with some extension to the nasal inferior visual field also.

a temporal visual field defect, but can also involve the nasal visual field (Figs 7.3 and 7.9).

Hydrocephalus

The optic chiasm is situated in the anteroinfero region of the third ventricle. An enlarged third ventricle due to raised intracranial pressure may press on the superior aspect of the chiasm resulting in a visual deficit of the inferior quadrants initially

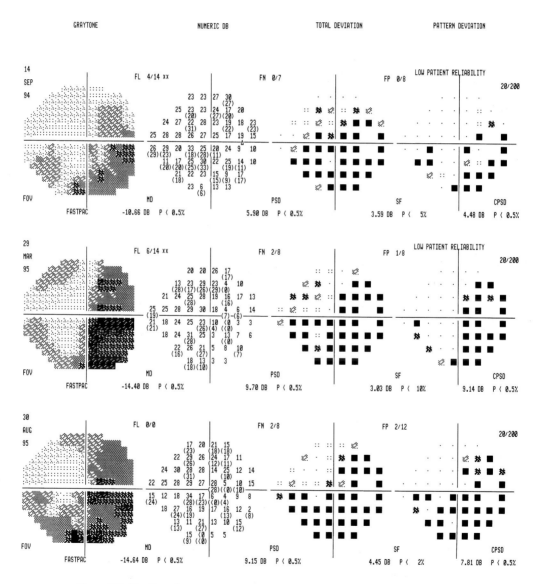

Figure 7.9 (Continued)

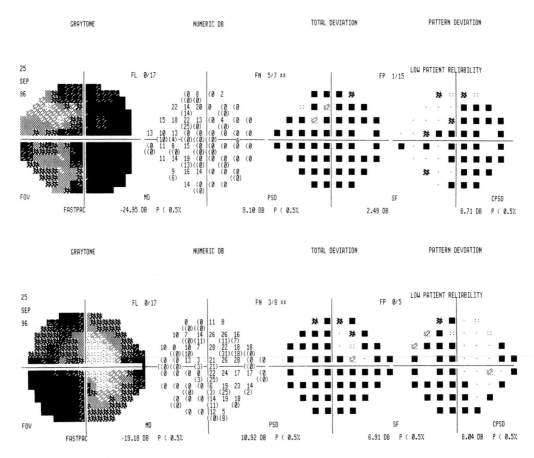

Figure 7.10 Humphrey perimeter visual field assessment: hydrocephalus. There is severe impairment of visual field, but particularly loss in the temporal visual field as evident on the pattern deviation plot and corrected pattern standard deviation plot. Note the decibel values for the bitemporal areas of the visual fields.

(Walsh & Hoyt 1982). The visual field loss can be more severe, particularly if there is papilloedema of the optic disc, thus giving rise to visual field defects of this part of the optic nerve in addition (Fig. 7.10).

Multiple sclerosis

This may commence with a central scotoma which progresses to hemianopic scotoma (Boldt *et al.* 1963).

Pituitary adenoma

Bitemporal visual field defects are classically associated with optic chiasm compression (Trobe 1974). The inferonasal retinal nerve fibres cross low and anteriorly, and

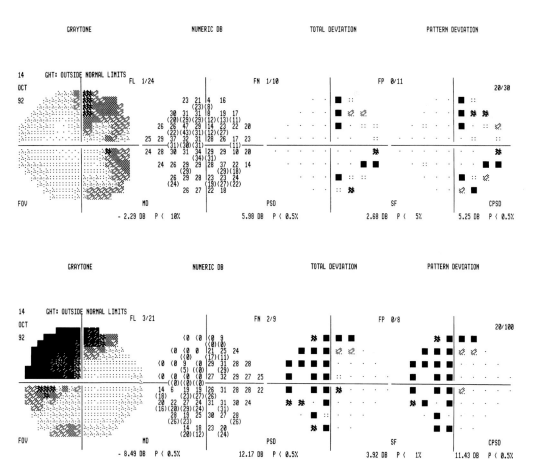

Figure 7.11 Humphrey perimeter visual field assessment: pituitary adenoma. There is superior temporal visual field impairment (left greater than right) due to involvement of the inferior retinal nerve fibres first. Note the decibel values and probability plots.

therefore are most vulnerable to damage from expanding sellar lesions, typically pituitary adenomas.

In about 80% of normal subjects the optic chiasm lies directly above the sella. As the tumour grows upwards it splays the anterior chiasmal notch and compresses the crossing inferonasal fibres, causing a defect in the upper visual field (Figs 7.5 and 7.11). With further tumour extension, the defect progresses in an anticlockwise direction in the left eye and clockwise in the right eye to involve the lower visual field.

Compression of the optic chiasm may be asymmetrical, thus causing an asymmetrical visual field defect such that temporal visual field loss is present in one eye but the other eye can have very little involvement (Fig. 7.12). With extensive compression of the optic chiasm there can be substantial loss of visual field (Fig. 7.13).

In approximately 10% of normal subjects, the optic chiasm is situated more anteriorly over the tuberculum sellae – prefixed (Walsh and Hoyt 1982). In this

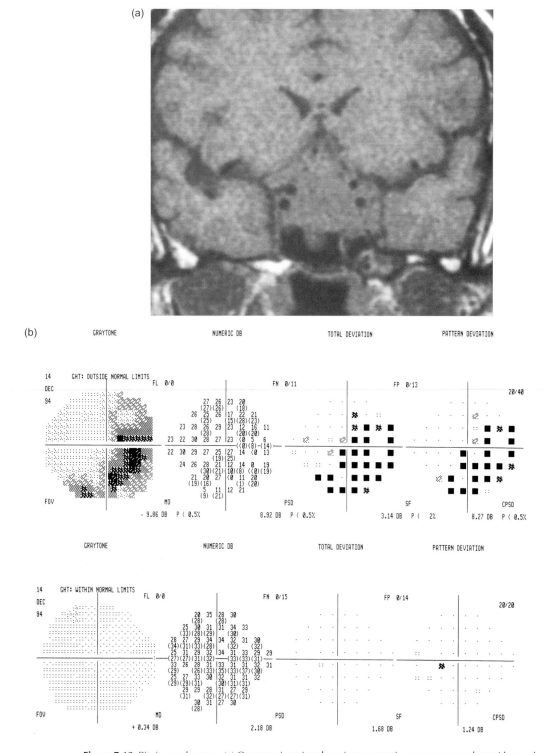

Figure 7.12 Pituitary adenoma. (a) On neuroimaging there is an extensive tumour mass, but with mostly lateral expansion and asymmetrical compression of the optic chiasm. (b) On visual field assessment there is right temporal visual field loss (inferior greater than superior, which is atypical but probably reflects the unusual expansion pattern of the tumour). The left eye result is normal.

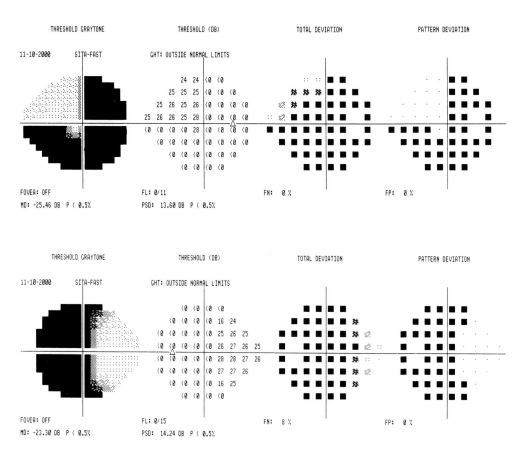

Figure 7.13 Humphrey perimeter visual field assessment: pituitary adenoma. There is complete bilateral temporal visual field loss and also nasal visual field loss. Note the decibel values and probability plots.

situation, pituitary tumours may compress the optic tract first, resulting in homonymous defects (Trobe 1974; Fig. 7.14). Elkington (1968) reported that homonymous hemianopia is uncommon, but is particularly associated with large and extensive tumours.

In 10% of cases, a postfixed optic chiasm occurs where the optic chiasm is located more posteriorly over the dorsum sellae. Suprasellar extension of a pituitary tumour will therefore compress the optic nerves (Trobe 1974; Manor *et al.* 1980). Nasal field loss caused by pituitary apoplexy is also documented (Manor *et al.* 1980; Rowe *et al.* 1995); the haemorrhage is thought to be responsible for the subsequent visual field deficit.

Manor *et al.*(1980) have reported monocular superior nasal loss and postulate an impaired circulation in the prechiasmal arterial anastomotic network. A generalised reduction in sensitivity may also be seen (Fig. 7.15) but a temporal preference is usual, even with this reduction in sensitivity (Fig. 7.16).

A paracentral scotoma in the superior temporal quadrant may represent a very early involvement of nasal retinal fibres by a tumour just extending to the optic

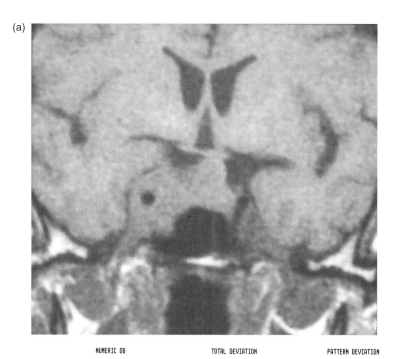

(a)

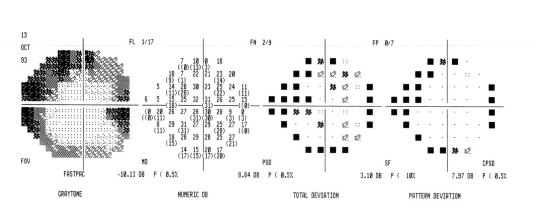

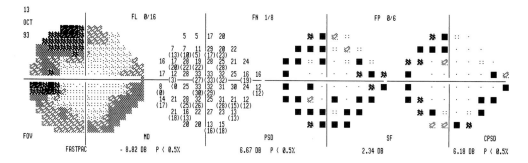

Figure 7.14 Pituitary adenoma. (a) On neuroimaging there is lateral expansion of the tumour. Superior expansion is asymmetrical and can be clearly seen to impinge on the posterior optic chiasm/optic tract. (b) On visual field assessment there is slight right temporal visual field loss, but predominantly superior nasal visual field loss; there is predominantly left superior temporal visual field loss. This reflects the atypical compression of the visual pathway by the tumour.

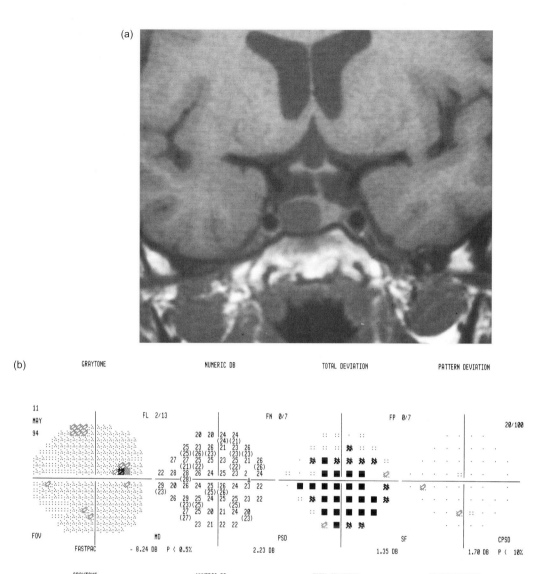

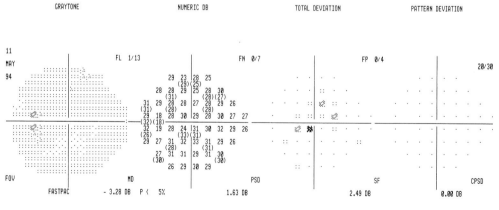

Figure 7.15 Pituitary adenoma. (a) On neuroimaging there is a small localised mass. (b) On visual field assessment there is reduced sensitivity across the right visual field with mild reduced central sensitivity in the left eye.

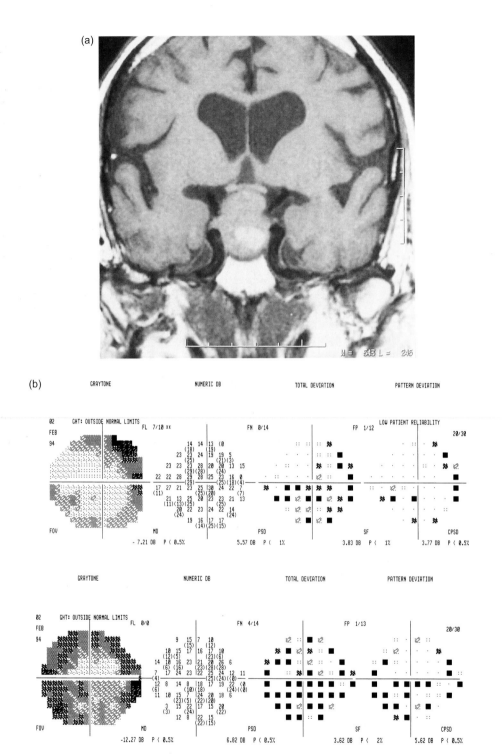

Figure 7.16 Pituitary adenoma. (a) On neuroimaging there is a large mass evident, but with a gap between the superior aspect of the tumour extension and the optic chiasm. The increased signal within the tumour mass represents a haemorrhage. (b) On visual field assessment there is reduced sensitivity in the right eye, particularly in the temporal and inferior nasal visual field as seen on the probability plots. The left eye has reduced sensitivity across the visual field, but the temporal visual field impairment is identified on the corrected pattern standard deviation plot.

(a)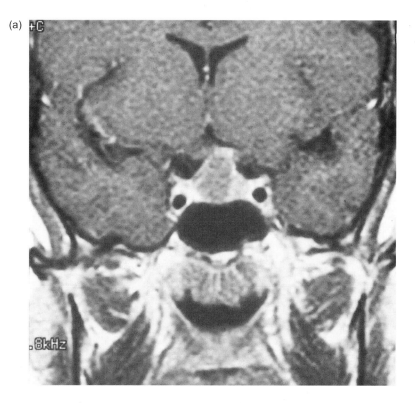

Figure 7.17 Pituitary adenoma. (a) On neuroimaging a small mass can be seen that just extends to the optic chiasm. (b) On visual field assessment there is a couple of spurious points involved in the right eye on the corrected pattern standard deviation plot. In the left eye there is a scotoma in the superior temporal visual field which is evident on the probability plots. Both right and left eye results are normal on follow-up after neurosurgery to remove the tumour.

chiasm (Fig. 7.17; Rowe *et al.* 1995). Junctional scotomas are a rarely documented field defect and are also described as an early feature of chiasmal compression (Bird 1972).

At times, visual field results will provide no specific information that an abnormality exists and will appear normal in most respects. However, the presence of at least three edge points (cluster) even when only mildly involved (Fig. 7.18) can be a give-away to the presence of pathology.

Vascular abnormalities

Nasal visual field defects (Fig. 7.6) may also be caused by arterial aneurysms. The internal carotid arteries are closely related to the optic nerves and optic chiasm, as is the precommunicating portion of the anterior cerebral artery. An aneurysm involving either of these arteries can therefore compress both the optic nerve (Mitts & McQueen 1965) and the optic chiasm. A dilatation of an internal carotid aneurysm

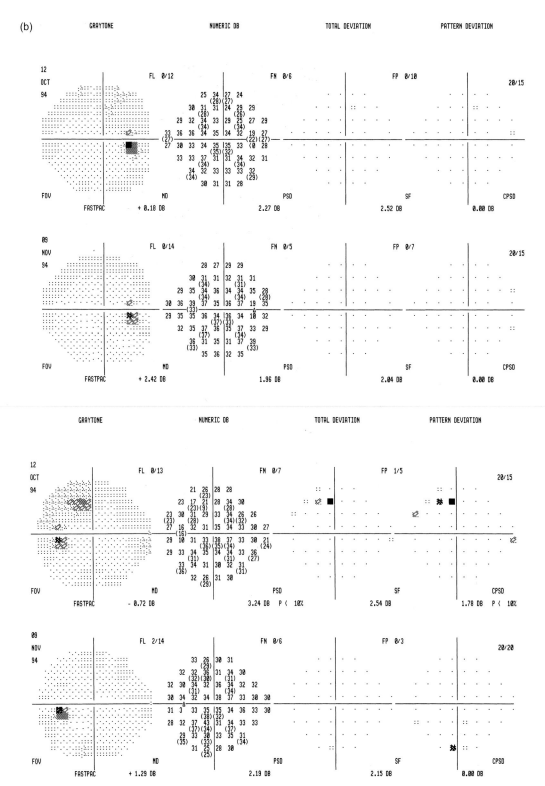

Figure 7.17 (Continued)

(a)

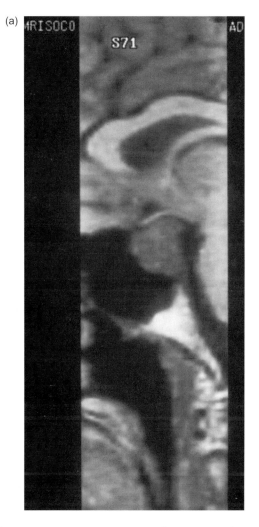

Figure 7.18 Pituitary adenoma. (a) On neuroimaging a small mass is seen that just extends to the optic chiasm but does not appear to impinge directly on the optic chiasm. (b) On visual field assessment the right eye result is normal. However, the left eye result shows four edge points involved in the temporal visual field which are evident on the corrected pattern standard deviation plot.

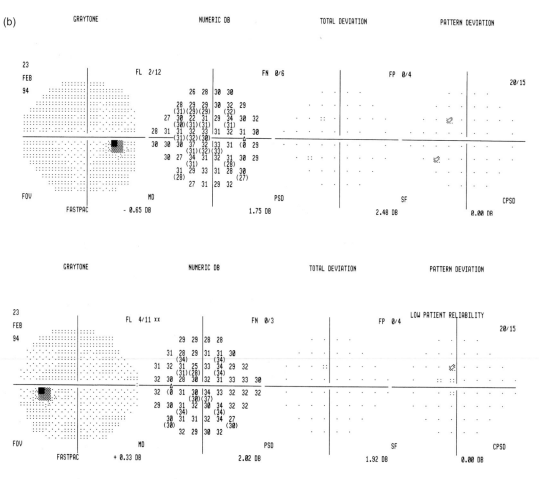

Figure 7.18 (Continued)

may cause lateral compression of the optic chiasm. The field defect is usually unilateral, but may be bilateral with large aneurysms or bilateral carotid aneurysms.

Binasal field loss is most probably due to pressure affecting the lateral aspects of the optic nerves rather than the lateral aspects of the optic chiasm (Walsh & Hoyt 1982).

Choice of visual field assessment

Generally, central visual field programmes will appropriately plot visual field loss, with optic chiasm lesions particularly, as the macular fibres also cross at the optic chiasm. However, peripheral visual field programmes should be undertaken if any doubt exists over the results of a central visual field programme or where full documentation of the entire visual field is required. Peripheral visual field assessment should be considered where there is a suspicion of junctional scotoma with temporal visual field loss in the fellow eye. Careful attention must be paid to the vertical meridian.

References

Bergland R, Ray BS (1969) Arterial supply of human optic chiasm. *Journal of Neurosurgery*, **31**: 327

Bergland RM, Ray BS, Torack RM (1968) Anatomical variations in the pituitary gland and adjacent structures in 225 human autopsy cases. *Journal of Neurosurgery*, **28**: 93

Bird AC (1972) Field loss due to lesions at the anterior angle of the chiasm. *Proceedings of the Royal Society of Medicine*, **65**: 519

Boldt HA, Armin FH, Tourtellette WW, De-Jong RN (1963) Retrochiasmal visual field defects from multiple sclerosis. *Archives of Neurology*, **8**: 565

Chamlin M, Davidoff LM, Feiring EH (1955) Ophthalmologic changes produced by pituitary tumors. *American Journal of Ophthalmology*, 40: 353

Drachman DA (1966) See-saw nystagmus. *Journal of Neurology, Neurosurgery and Psychiatry*, **29**: 356

Elkington SG (1968) Pituitary adenoma. Preoperative symptomatology in a series of 260 patients. *British Journal of Ophthalmology*, **52**: 322

Glaser JS, Hoyt WF, Corbett J (1971) Visual morbidity with chiasmal glioma. *Archives of Ophthalmology*, 85: 3

Glaser JS (1978) Neuro-ophthalmology, In: *Clinical Opthamology* (ed. TD Duane). Hagerstown, Harper and Row, pp. 135–151.

Hershenfeld SA, Sharpe JA (1993) Monocular temporal hemianopia. *British Journal of Ophthalmology*, 77: 424

Horton JC (1997) Wilbrand's knee of the primate optic chiasm is an artefact of monocular enucleation. *Transactions of American Ophthalmic Society*, 95: 579

Hughes B (1958) Blood supply of the optic nerve and chiasm and its clinical significance. *British Journal of Ophthalmology*, 42: 106

Kearns TP, Rucker CW (1958) Arcuate defects in the visual fields due to chromophobe adenoma of the pituitary gland. *American Journal of Ophthalmology*, 45: 505

Kirkham TH (1972) The ocular symptomatology of pituitary tumours. *Proceedings of the Royal Society of Medicine*, **65**: 517

Manor RS, Ouaknine GE, Matz S, Shalit MN (1980) Nasal visual field loss with intracranial lesions of the optic nerve pathways. *American Journal of Ophthalmology*, **90**: 1

Mitts MG, McQueen JD (1965) Visual loss associated with fusiform enlargement of the intracranial portion of the internal carotid artery. *Journal of Neurosurgery*, **23**: 33

Moller PM, Hvid-Hansen O (1970) Chiasmal visual fields. *Acta Ophthalmologica*, **48**: 678

Rowe F, Thompson C, Webster AR (1995) Incidence of bitemporal hemianopic visual field defects in pituitary tumours. In: *Transactions of 8th International Orthoptic Congress*, p. 279

Rowe F (1996) Visual disturbances in chiasmal lesions. *British Orthoptic Journal*, **53**: 1

Rowe FJ (1998) Esterman driving tests using Humphrey automated perimetry. *British Orthoptic Journal*, **55**: 57–65

Schiefer U, Isbert M, Mikoloschek E, Mildenberger I, Krapp E, Schiller J, Thanos S, Hart W (2004) Distribution of scotoma pattern related to chiasmal lesions with special reference to anterior junction syndrome. *Graefes Archives of Clinical and Experimental Ophthalmology*, **242**: 468

Trobe JD (1974) Chromophobe adenoma presenting with a hemianopic temporal arcuate scotoma. *American Journal of Ophthalmology*, **77**: 388

Walsh FB, Gass JD (1960) Concerning the optic chiasm. Selected pathologic involvement and clinical problems. The de Schweinitz lecture. *American Journal of Ophthalmology*, **50**: 1031

Walsh FB, Hoyt WF (1982) *Clinical Neuro-Ophthalmology*, 4th edn, Vol. 1 (ed. N Miller). Baltimore, Williams and Wilkins; pp. 60–68, 119–129

Wilbrand HL (1926) Schema des verlaufs der sehnervenfasern durch das chiasma. *Zeitschrift für Augenheilkunde*, **59**: 135

Wilson P, Falconer MA (1968) Patterns of visual failure with pituitary tumours. Clinical and radiological correlations. *British Journal of Ophthalmology*, **52**: 94

Wollschlaeger PB, Wollschlaeger G, Ide CH, Hart WM (1971) Arterial blood supply of the human optic chiasm and surrounding structures. *Annals of Ophthalmology*, **3**: 862

Wybar K (1977) Presenting ocular features. *Proceedings of the Royal Society of Medicine*, **70**: 307

Further reading

Adler FH, Kaufman PL (eds) (2002) *Adler's Physiology of the Eye. Clinical Application*, 10th edn. St Louis, Mosby

Barber AN, Ronstrom GN, Muelling RJ Jr (1954) Development of the visual pathway: optic chiasm. *Archives of Ophthalmology*, **52**: 447

Brouwer B, Zeeman WPC (1925) Experimental anatomical investigation concerning the projection of the retina on the primary optic centres in apes. *Journal of Neurology and Psychiatry*, **6**: 1

Brouwer B, Zeeman WPC (1926) The projection of the retina in the primary optic neuron in monkeys. *Brain*, **49**: 1

Carmel PW, Antunes JL, Chang CH (1982) Craniopharyngiomas in children. *Neurosurgery*, **11**: 382

Cope VZ (1916) The pituitary fossa and the methods of surgical approach thereto. *British Journal of Surgery*, **4**: 107

Corbett JJ (1986) Neuro-ophthalmologic complications of hydrocephalus and shunting procedures. *Seminars on Neurology*, **6**: 111

Eldevik OP, Blaivas M, Gabrielson TO, Hald JK, Chandler WF (1996) Craniopharyngioma: radiologic and histologic findings and recurrence. *American Journal of Neuroradiology*, **17**: 1427

Fletcher WA, Imes RK, Hoyt WF (1986) Chiasmal gliomas: appearance and long-term changes demonstrated by computerized tomography. *Journal of Neurosurgery*, **65**: 154

Glaser JS (1967) The nasal visual field. *Archives of Ophthalmology*, **77**: 358

Gregorius FK, Hepler RS, Stern WE (1975) Loss and recovery of vision with suprasellar meningioma. *Journal of Neurosurgery*, **42**: 69

Heinz GW, Nunery WR, Grossman CB (1994) Traumatic chiasmal syndrome associated with midline basilar skull fractures. *American Journal of Ophthalmology*, **117**: 90

Hoyt WF (1969) Correlative functional anatomy of the optic chiasm. *Clinical Neurosurgery*, **17**: 189

Hoyt WF, Luis O (1962) The primate chiasm; details of visual fibre organisation studied by silver impregnation techniques. *Archives of Ophthalmology*, **68**: 94

Ikeda H, Yoshimoto T (1995) Visual disturbances in patients with pituitary adenoma. *Acta Neurologica Scandinavica*, **92**: 157

Kanski J (2003) *Clinical Ophthalmology. A Systematic Approach.* 5th edn. London, Butterworth Heinemann

Kanski J (2004) *Clinical Ophthalmology. A Synopsis.* London. Butterworth Heinemann/ Elsevier Science

Kupfer C, Chumbley L, de Downer JC (1967) Quantitative histology of optic nerve, optic tract and lateral geniculate nucleus of man. *Journal of Anatomy*, **101**: 393

Lindgren E (1957) Radiologic examination of the brain and spinal cord. *Acta Radiologica Suppl.* **151**: 1

McFadzean RM, Doyle D, Rampling R, Teasdale E, Teasdale G (1991) Pituitary apoplexy and its effect on vision. *Neurosurgery*, **29**: 669

McLone DG, Raimondi AJ, Naidich TP (1982) Craniopharyngiomas. *Child's Brain*, **8**: 188

Marcus RC, Blazeski R, Godement P, Mason CA (1995) Retinal axon divergence in the optic chiasm: uncrossed axons diverge from crossed axons within a midline glial specialisation. *Journal of Neuroscience*, **15**: 3716

O'Connell JEA, DuBoulay EPGH (1973) Binasal hemianopia. *Journal of Neurology, Neurosurgery and Psychiatry*, **36**: 697

Olivero WC, Lister R, Elwood PW (1995) The natural history and growth rate of asymptomatic meningiomas: a review of 60 patients. *Journal of Neurosurgery*, **83**: 222

Olver J, Cassidy L (2005) *Opthalmology at a Glance.* Oxford, Blackwell Publishing

Perlmutter D, Rhoton AL (1976) Microsurgical anatomy of the anterior cerebral–anterior communicating recurrent artery complex. *Journal of Neurosurgery*, **45**: 259

Polyak SL (1958) *The Vertebrate Visual System*, Chicago, University of Chicago Press

Rhoton AL, Harris FS, Renn WH (1977) Microsurgical anatomy of the sellar region and cavernous sinus. *Neuro Ophthalmology*, **9**: 1

Rolih CA, Ober P (1993) Pituitary apoplexy. *Endocrinology Metabolism Clinics of North America*, **22**: 291

Rucker CW (1958) The concept of a semidecussation of the optic nerves. *Archives of Ophthalmology*, **59**: 159

Savino PJ, Glaser JS, Schatz NJ (1980) Traumatic chiasmal syndrome. *Neurology*, **30**: 963

Schaeffer JP (1924) Some points in the regional anatomy of the optic pathway with specific reference to tumors of the hypophysis cerebri and resulting ocular changes. *Anatomical Record*, **28**: 243

Schweinitz GDE (1923) The Bowman lecture. Concerning certain ocular aspects of pituitary body disorders, mainly exclusive of the usual central and peripheral hemianopia. *Transactions of the Ophthalmological Societies of the UK*, **43**: 12

Sinclair AHH, Dott NM (1931) Hydrocephalus simulating tumour in the production of chiasmal and other parahypophysial lesions. *Transactions of the Ophthalmological Societies of the UK*, **51**: 232

Snell RS, Lemp MA (1998) *Clinical Anatomy of the Eye*, 2nd edn. Oxford, Blackwell Publishing

Spector RH, Glaser JS, Schatz NJ (1980) Demyelinative chiasmal lesions. *Archives of Neurology*, **37**: 757

Traquair HM (1916) The anatomic relations of the hypophysis and chiasma. *Ophthalmoscope*, **14**: 562

Unsold R, Hoyt WF (1980) Band atrophy of the optic nerve. *Archives of Ophthalmology*, **98**: 1637

Waespe W, Haenny P (1987) Bitemporal hemianopia due to chiasmal optic neuritis. *Neuro Ophthalmology*, **7**: 69

Chapter 8

Optic tract

Anatomy*

The retinal nerve fibres, after having passed through the optic chiasm, travel posteriorly toward the lateral geniculate body by way of the optic tracts. The optic tracts sweep laterally from the optic chiasm, passing around the ventral portion of the midbrain and encircling the hypothalamus posteriorly. The majority of retinal nerve fibres terminate in the lateral geniculate body. A smaller number continue to the pretectal area (pupillary reflexes).

Each optic tract contains crossed nasal retinal fibres that originate in the contralateral nasal hemiretina and uncrossed temporal retinal fibres that originate in the ipsilateral temporal hemiretina. The nerve fibres from corresponding retinal areas are not, however, paired straight away in the optic tract.

As the crossed and uncrossed retinal nerve fibres, corresponding to an entire hemifield, eventually converge, the crossed nasal inferior retinal nerve fibres become related to uncrossed temporal inferior retinal nerve fibres, and crossed superior retinal nerve fibres become related to uncrossed superior retinal nerve fibres. The macular fibres come to lie superolaterally. The nerve fibres from both superior retinas are located superomedially and the nerve fibres from both inferior retinas are located inferolaterally. The retinotopic map is tilted in the optic tracts so that the macula is represented dorsally, inferior retina laterally and superior retina medially.

The optic tracts obtain their blood supply via a pial plexus. This is continuous anteriorly with that of the optic chiasm and fed partly from the posterior communicating artery but mainly from the anterior choroidal artery. It is also supplied by branches of the middle cerebral artery (Francois *et al.* 1956).

---

*This anatomy section is intended as a brief description only. If required, further detail should be sought from appropriate textbooks – see Further reading. The anatomy and pathology sections, in combination, provide a background to the part of the visual pathway covered in this chapter so that the relevant visual field defects can be considered and interpreted appropriately.

Pathology*

Optic tract defects are uncommon, and lesions of the optic tract are similar to those causing damage to the optic chiasm. Typically these include pituitary adenomas with posterior extension, craniopharyngioma and other parasellar tumours, demyelination and vascular abnormalities. Most commonly, optic tract defects result from a compressive tumour extending posteriorly from the optic chiasm area, or trauma at the time of surgical removal of the tumour.

Less common causes of optic tract pathology include inflammatory conditions (such as multiple sclerosis and sarcoid), migraine, trauma and radiotherapy.

Craniopharyngioma

These are slow growing tumours arising from the vestigal remnants of Rathke's pouch along the pituitary stalk (Fig. 8.1). The tumour compresses the tract from above and ventrally.

Meningioma

Meningiomas that involve the optic tract may arise from the tuberculum sellae or lesser wing of sphenoid and are slow growing. These tumours typically affect middle aged women and often cause hyperosmosis which can be seen on a plain skull X-ray.

Pituitary tumours

In approximately 10% of normal subjects, the optic chiasm is situated more anteriorly over the tuberculum sellae – prefixed (Walsh & Hoyt 1982). In this situation, pituitary tumours may compress the optic tract first, resulting in homonymous defects (Trobe 1974; see Fig. 7.14).

Trauma

In trauma, acceleration/deceleration injuries are caused by the movement of the brain relative to the skull. The impact to the head produces a rapid movement of both the skull and brain in the direction of the force. The brain lags behind the faster moving skull resulting in high pressure in the brain at the area of impact and low pressure at the counter pole. Shock waves are induced and are transmitted through the brain causing damage to the visual pathway (diffuse axonal injury or shearing injuries). Intracranial effects include effects from haemorrhage or ischaemia.

---

*This pathology section is provided as a summary of possible disease processes but by its nature cannot be all inclusive. The reader is directed towards other appropriate textbooks for further detail – see Further reading.

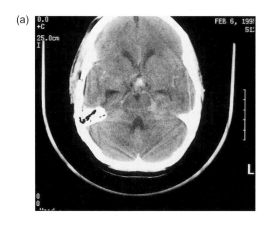

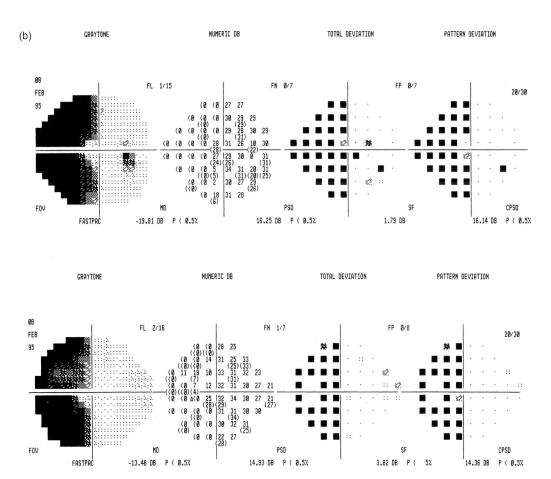

Figure 8.1 Craniopharyngioma. (a) On neuroimaging a mass lesion is evident centrally in the middle cranial fossa. (b) On visual field assessment there is an incongruous left homonymous hemianopia. Note the decibel values in particular and the probability plots. Central vision is retained.

Vascular abnormalities

Vascular lesions may include a cerebrovascular accident (stroke) with involvement of the anterior choroidal artery, middle cerebral artery or posterior cerebral artery. Stroke is defined as a clinical syndrome consisting of rapidly developing signs of focal (or global) disturbance of cerebral function, lasting more than 24 hours or leading to death, with no apparent cause other than of vascular origin (World Health Organisation). There are two broad categories: (a) cerebral infarct as a result of a temporary or permanent occlusion of a feeding artery (extra- or intracranially) and

(a)

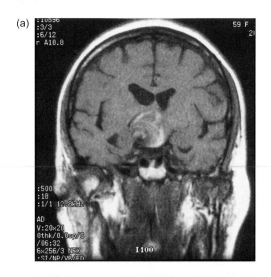

(b)

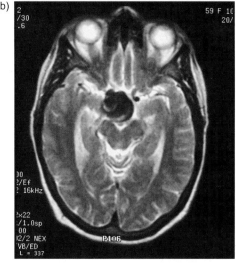

Figure 8.2 Internal carotid artery aneurysm. (a,b) On neuroimaging note the mass effect of the aneurysm centrally. (c) On visual field assessment there is a left homonymous hemianopia which is congruous.

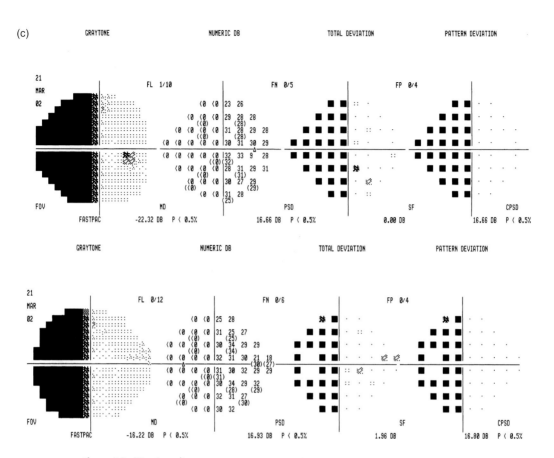

Figure 8.2 (Continued)

accounts for about 80% of strokes (Bamford 1992) and (b) cerebral haemorrhage due to a rupture of an abnormal artery (aneurysm or arteriovenous malformation) or arteriole in the brain parenchyma.

Optic tract involvement may also occur with suprasellar aneurysms (Fig. 8.2).

Associated signs and symptoms*

General signs

A lesion of the optic tract may damage the ipsilateral cerebral peduncle and give rise to mild contralateral pyramidal signs. Other associated abnormalities are unusual, but may include endocrine disturbances because of interference with hypothalamic function and memory impairment from temporal lobe involvement (Bender & Bodis Wollner 1978).

---

*This section on associated signs and symptoms is provided so that the practitioner is aware of additional information that can be considered in conjunction with the visual field defect to aid differential diagnosis and localisation of pathology.

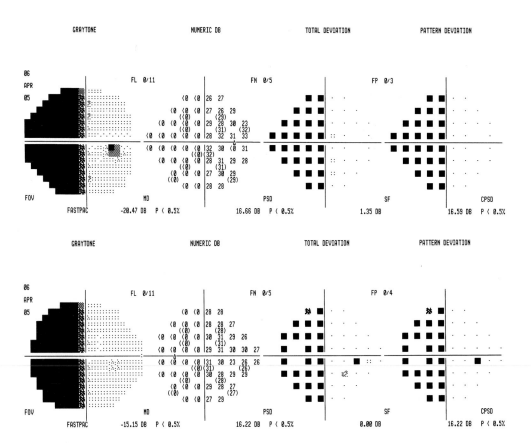

Figure 8.3 Humphrey perimeter visual field assessment: migraine. There is a congruous complete left homonymous hemianopia.

Although they do not secrete hormones, craniopharyngiomas may interfere with hypothalamic function, and in children they may cause pituitary dwarfism, diabetes insipidus, delayed sexual development and occasionally obesity. Presentation in childhood is commonly related to hydrocephalus.

Pituitary adenomas occur with and without clinically manifest endocrine activity. Pituitary hormones include adrenocorticotrophic hormone (ACTH), thyroid stimulating hormone (TSH), luteinising hormone (LH), follicle stimulating hormone (FSH), somatotropin (STH) and prolactin. Ensuing non-ocular problems include Cushing syndrome, acromegaly, gigantism, infertility, amenorrhoea and galactorrhoea.

Optic atrophy

Because the cell bodies of all nerve fibres in the optic tract are the retinal ganglion cells, optic atrophy may result when these fibres are damaged due to retrograde degeneration (Paul & Hoyt 1976).

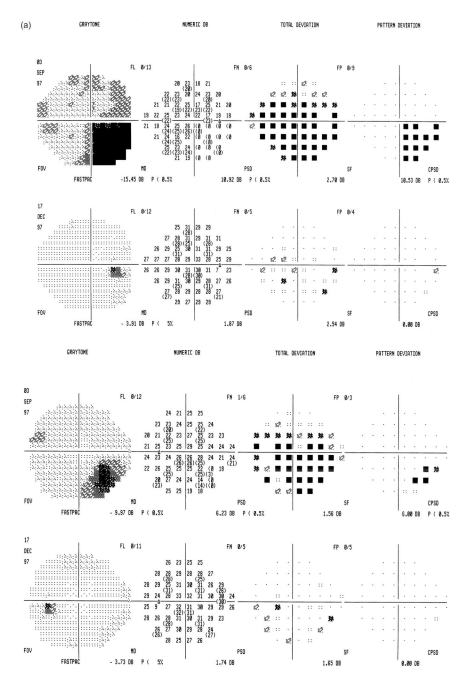

Figure 8.4 Humphrey perimeter visual field assessment: meningioma. (a) There is a mostly incongruous right homonymous hemianopia. The right eye shows temporal visual field loss, particularly in the inferior visual field, with inferior nasal loss also (note decibel values and probability plots). The left eye shows right inferior nasal visual field loss. Following surgery there is a vast improvement in visual field function which is evident also on the change analysis (b) with centralisation of the boxplot and increase in global indices.

(b)

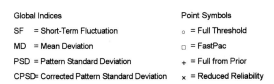

Global Indices

SF   = Short-Term Fluctuation

MD   = Mean Deviation

PSD = Pattern Standard Deviation

CPSD= Corrected Pattern Standard Deviation

Point Symbols

o = Full Threshold

□ = FastPac

+ = Full from Prior

x = Reduced Reliability

Figure 8.4 (Continued)

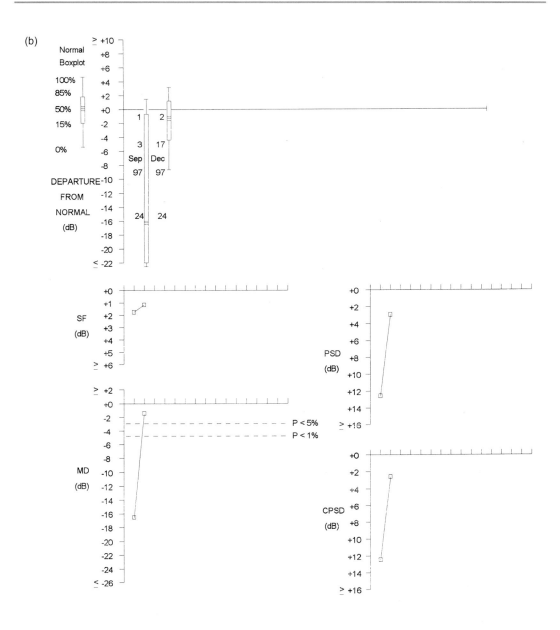

(b)

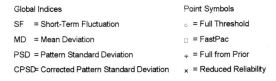

Global Indices

SF   = Short-Term Fluctuation
MD = Mean Deviation
PSD = Pattern Standard Deviation
CPSD= Corrected Pattern Standard Deviation

Point Symbols

o = Full Threshold
□ = FastPac
+ = Full from Prior
x = Reduced Reliability

Figure 8.4 (Continued)

Pupil abnormalities

The optic tracts contain retinal nerve fibres that subserve both visual and pupillary functions. The retinal nerve fibres terminate in the lateral geniculate body, but the pupillary nerve fibres leave the optic tract prior to the lateral geniculate body, project through the brachium of the superior colliculus and terminate in the pretectal nucleus. An optic tract lesion may therefore produce an afferent pupillary conduction defect. Typically, the pupillary light reaction is normal when the unaffected hemiretina is stimulated and absent when the involved hemiretina is stimulated. However, in practice, this Wernicke's hemianopic pupillary reaction is difficult to elicit.

The relative afferent pupillary defect is usually in the eye with the temporal visual field loss. This is attributed to the greater size of the temporal visual field and a slightly larger number of axons from the nasal than temporal retina (Bell & Thompson 1978).

Visual field defects

In previous chapters, visual field loss has been described in relation to the pathological categories causing the visual field deficit. However, as various pathological categories tend to cause similar types of visual field loss in optic tract disease, it is the visual field loss that will be described in categories in this section.

Visual field defects are characterised by the marked incongruity of the field defect in association with an afferent pupillary defect on the same side as the hemianopia, from damage to the pupillary nerve fibres in the optic tract, and bilateral optic disc pallor.

Congruous visual field loss

With marked involvement of the optic tract by pathological lesions, a complete homonymous hemianopia will be noted which has no localising value (Fig. 8.3).

Incongruous visual field loss

Partial lesions of the optic tract will cause contralateral homonymous visual field defects, but the incomplete pairing of the retinal nerve fibres of the two eyes results in incongruity. Marked incongruity indicates an optic tract lesion, since lesions of the optic radiations tend to cause only mild incongruity and visual cortex lesions are highly congruous.

Incongruity can vary considerably, from marked dissimilarity of the two eyes (Fig. 8.4) to less dissimilarity (Fig. 8.1). Sometimes the visual fields will appear congruous, but careful examination of the sensitivities of the visual fields of either eye will reveal minor dissimilarities (Fig. 8.2).

The combination of optic atrophy, relative afferent pupillary defect and visual field incongruity are important to recognise in a patient with homonymous hemifield defects because the differential diagnosis of optic tract lesions differs greatly from that of lesions of the optic radiations or striate visual cortex. While visual field defects related to optic radiation or striate visual cortex lesions result from vascular disease and other intracerebral pathology, most optic tract lesions are compressive extrinsic masses. Elkington (1968) reported that homonymous hemianopia as a result of an optic tract lesion is uncommon, but is particularly associated with large and extensive tumours such as compression from a pituitary adenoma with a prefixed optic chiasm.

Choice of visual field assessment

Central visual field assessment is usually sufficient to detect most field defects due to pathology of the optic tract. If pathology is suspected or known but there are no visual field defects centrally, a peripheral visual field test may demonstrate a homonymous loss of visual field in the peripheral field of vision. Peripheral visual field programmes should be undertaken if any doubt exists over the results of a central visual field programme or where full documentation of the entire visual field is required. Careful attention must be paid to the vertical meridia.

References

Bamford J (1992) Clinical examination in the diagnosis and subclassification of stroke. *Lancet*, **339**: 400

Bell RA, Thompson HS (1978) Relative afferent pupillary defect in optic tract hemianopias. *American Journal of Ophthalmology*, **85**: 538

Bender MB, Bodis Wollner I (1978) Visual dysfunctions in optic tract lesions. *Annals of Neurology*, **3**: 187

Elkington SG (1968) Pituitary adenoma. Preoperative symptomatology in a series of 260 patients. *British Journal of Opthalmology*, **52**: 322

Francois J, Neetans A, Collette JM (1956) Vascularisation of the optic pathway IV. Optic tract and geniculate body. *British Journal of Ophthalmology*, **40**: 341

Paul TO, Hoyt WF (1976) Fundoscopic appearance of papilloedema with optic tract atrophy. *Archives of Ophthalmology*, **94**: 467

Trobe JD (1974) Chromophobe adenoma presenting with a hemianopic temporal arcuate scotoma. *American Journal of Ophthalmology*, **77**: 388

Walsh FB, Hoyt WF (1982) Clinical Neuro-Opthalmology, 4th edn. Vol. 1 (ed. N Miller) Baltimore, Williams and Wilkins; pp.60–68, 119–129

World Health Organisation. www.who.int/en

Further reading

Adler FH, Kaufman PL (eds) (2002) *Adler's Physiology of the Eye. Clinical Application*, 10th edn. St Louis, Mosby

Jacobson DM (1997) The localizing value of a quadrantanopia. *Archives of Neurology*, **54**: 401

Kanski J (2003) *Clinical Opthalmology. A Systematic Approach*, 5th edn. London, Butterworth Heinemann

Kanski J (2004) *Clinical Opthalmology. A Synopsis*. London, Butterworth Heinemann/Elsevier Science

Newman SA, Miller NR (1983) The optic tract syndrome; neuro-ophthalmologic considerations. *Archives of Ophthalmology*, **101**: 1241

Olver J, Cassidy L (2005) *Opthalmology at a Glance*. Oxford, Blackwell Publishing

Plant GT, Kermode AG, Turano G, Moseley IF, Miller DH, MacManus DG, Halliday AM, McDonald WI (1992) Symptomatic retrochiasmal lesions in multiple sclerosis. Clinical features, visual evoked potentials and magnetic resonance imaging. *Neurology*, **42**: 68

Savino PJ, Paris M, Schatz NJ, Orr LS, Corbett JJ (1978) Optic tract syndrome: a review of 21 patients. *Archives of Ophthalmology*, **96**: 656

Smith JL (1962) Homonymous hemianopia: a review of one hundred cases. *American Journal of Ophthalmology*, **54**: 616

Snell RS, Lemp MA (1998) *Clinical Anatomy of the Eye*, 2nd edn. Oxford, Blackwell Publishing

Wilbrand HL (1926) Schema des verlaufs der sehnervenfasern durch das chiasma. *Zeitschrift für Augenheilkunde* **59**: 135

Chapter 9

Lateral geniculate body

Anatomy*

The lateral geniculate body is a subnucleus of the thalamus. The lateral geniculate body (or nucleus) is located in the diencephalon lateral to the medial geniculate body and consists of a dorsal and ventral nucleus. The ventral nucleus is more primitive and has no visual function in man. The dorsal nucleus occupies the major portion of the lateral geniculate body and functions as the relay station for the primary afferent visual pathway.

The axons of retinal ganglion cells carrying visual impulses synapse in the lateral geniculate body (O'Leary et al. 1965). The lateral geniculate body is a triangular shaped structure with six horizontal domed layers containing segregated inputs from the two eyes (Clark 1932; Fig. 9.1).

The nerve fibres in the lateral geniculate body have a complicated arrangement. The nerve fibres rotate through an angle of 90 degrees. Consequently, superior or inferior retinal nerve fibres become displaced medially and laterally. This twist in the arrangement of visual fibres straightens again in the optic radiations so that, with the exception of the region of the lateral geniculate body, superior retinal nerve fibres remain relatively superior and inferior retinal nerve fibres remain relatively inferior throughout the visual pathway.

The central visual field is represented by all six cell layers of the lateral geniculate body (Kupfer 1962) while the remainder of the binocular field projects to only four layers. The ventral two layers are the magnocellular layers, whereas the other four layers are the parvocellular component. The macula is represented in a dorsal wedge, whereas the most peripheral fibres are located ventrally. Superior retinal fibres are in the medial horn and inferior retinal fibres are in the lateral horn. The monocular crescent is represented by one parvocellular and one magnocellular layer. Retinal nerve fibres from the temporal ipsilateral side synapse in layers 2, 3 and 5 while retinal nerve fibres from the nasal contralateral side synapse in layers 1, 4 and 6.

---

*This anatomy section is intended as a brief description only. If required, further detail should be sought from appropriate textbooks – see Further reading. The anatomy and pathology sections, in combination, provide a background to the part of the visual pathway covered in this chapter so that the relevant visual field defects can be considered and interpreted appropriately.

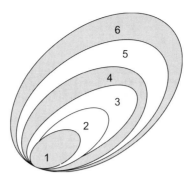

Figure 9.1 Lateral geniculate body structure. There are six layers in a domed shape with ipsilateral representation in layers 2, 3 and 5, and contralateral representation in layers 1, 4 and 6.

After synapse in the lateral geniculate body, corresponding nasal and temporal nerve fibres have the same representation in the optic radiation. The optic radiations arise from the dorsolateral surface of the lateral geniculate body.

The lateral geniculate body has a dual blood supply involving the anterior choroidal artery (branch of the internal carotid artery) and lateral choroidal artery (branch of the posterior cerebral artery). The anterior choroidal artery supplies both the lateral and medial aspects of the lateral geniculate body, and the lateral choroidal artery supplies the hilus and midzone (Abbie 1933; Francois *et al.* 1956).

Pathology*

Lesions of the lateral geniculate body are rare, but can be diagnosed from the clinical features and confirmed with magnetic resonance imaging scanning. Most lesions relate to cerebrovascular pathology, such as haemorrhage, infarction or arteriovenous malformation (Shacklett *et al.* 1984; Wada *et al.* 1999; Saeki *et al.* 2003). Specifically, occlusion of the anterior and lateral choroidal arteries will produce a lesion of the lateral geniculate body (Shacklett *et al.* 1984; Wada *et al.* 1999). An arteriovenous malformation is a developmental anomalous communication between the arterial and venous systems without intervening capillary beds. Blood is therefore shunted directly from the arteries to the venous circulation. Many malformations remain silent. However, there may be problems with associated haemorrhage or shunting of blood away from otherwise normal brain tissue.

The lateral geniculate body can also be involved in closed head injuries where nerve fibres from the visual pathway can be sheared and avulsion may occur at the lateral geniculate body. Very rarely, a small space-occupying lesion will involve the lateral geniculate body resulting in visual field deficit (Shacklett *et al.* 1984).

---

*This pathology section is provided as a summary of possible disease processes but by its nature cannot be all inclusive. The reader is directed towards other appropriate textbooks for further detail – see Further reading.

Optic atrophy

Lesions of the lateral geniculate body may result in optic disc atrophy due to retrograde degeneration of the retinal nerve fibres that synapse in the lateral geniculate body.

Pupil abnormalities

Visual field defects will occur with lesions of the lateral geniculate body but pupillary abnormalities (relative afferent pupillary defect) are not present as these fibres leave the optic tract before reaching the lateral geniculate body to pass to the pretectal nucleus via the superior brachium.

The presence of optic atrophy with homonymous visual field loss, but without a relative afferent pupillary defect, will aid differential diagnosis of a lesion of the lateral geniculate body from an optic tract lesion.

Visual field defects

A number of varying types of visual field defects may occur with lesions of the lateral geniculate body, dependent on the extent and nature of the lesion and the area of lateral geniculate body involved. Incongruous homonymous hemianopia may be noted (Gunderson & Hoyt 1971) similar to cases with optic tract lesions. Sectoral or wedge shaped hemianopias may also occur which reflect the vascular supply to the lateral geniculate body (division of anterior and lateral posterior choroidal arteries) (Shacklett *et al.* 1984).

Visual field defects will always involve central fixation due to the representation of the central retinal nerve fibres in all six layers of the lateral geniculate body, whereas monocular and binocular peripheral nerve fibres are distributed in varying layers of the lateral geniculate body (Fig. 9.2).

Retinal nerve fibres originating from inferior, central and superior retina are essentially located laterally, centrally and medially, respectively, in the lateral geniculate body (Saeki *et al.* 2003). With lateral choroidal ischaemia, the hilum and middle zone of the lateral geniculate body are affected, causing a wedge shaped visual defect straddling the horizontal meridian. With anterior choroidal ischaemia, the lateral and medial tips of the lateral geniculate body are involved, resulting in the reverse defect of loss of the superior and inferior aspects of the contralateral hemifield with sparing around the horizontal meridian.

The involvement of central fixation can aid differential diagnosis of a lateral geniculate body lesion from optic disc lesions which typically spare central fixation.

**This section on associated signs and symptoms is provided so that the practitioner is aware of additional information that can be considered in conjunction with the visual field defect to aid differential diagnosis and localisation of pathology.

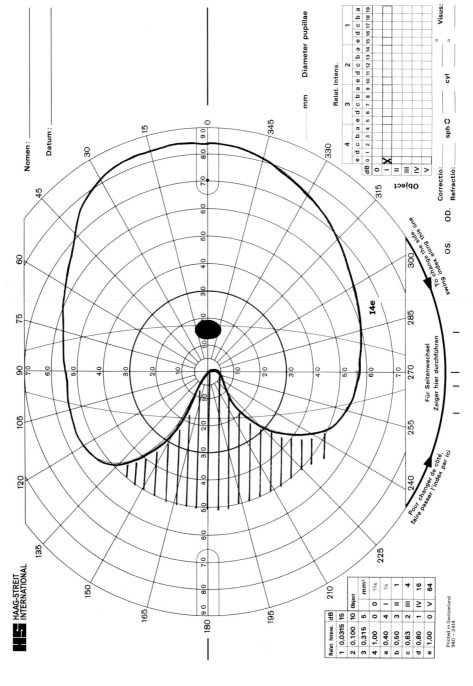

Figure 9.2 Goldmann perimeter visual field assessment: sector defect. There is an incongruous homonymous defect extending to central fixation.

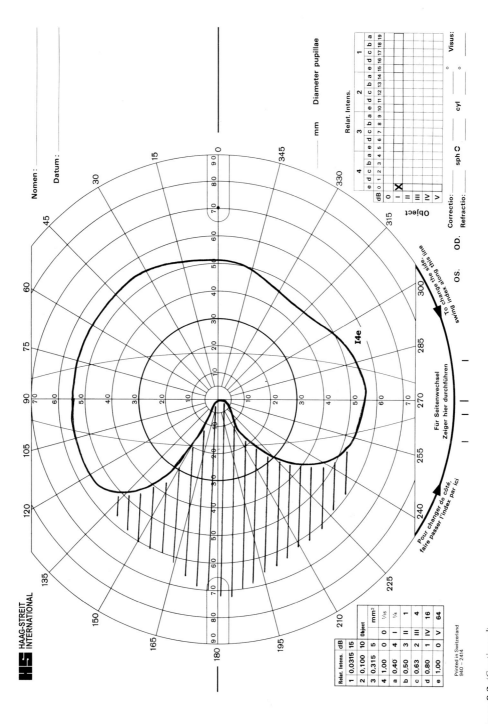

Figure 9.2 (Continued)

Choice of visual field assessment

Central visual field assessment is usually sufficient to detect most field defects due to pathology of the lateral geniculate body, particularly as central fixation is represented in all six layers of the nucleus. If pathology is suspected or known but there are no visual field defects centrally, a peripheral visual field test may demonstrate a homonymous loss of visual field peripherally. Peripheral visual field programmes should be undertaken if any doubt exists over the results of a central visual field programme or where full documentation of the entire visual field is required. Careful attention must be paid to central fixation.

References

Abbie AA (1933) The blood supply of LGB with note on morphology of choroidal arteries. *Journal of Anatomy*, **67**: 491

Clark WEL (1932) A morphological study of the lateral geniculate body. *British Journal of Ophthalmology*, **16**: 264

Francois J, Neetans A, Collette JM (1956) Vascularisation of the optic pathway IV. Optic tract and geniculate body. *British Journal of Ophthalmology*, **40**: 341

Gunderson CH, Hoyt WF (1971) Geniculate hemianopia: incongruous homonymous field defects in two patients with partial lesions of the lateral geniculate nucleus. *Journal of Neurology, Neurosurgery and Psychiatry*, **34**: 1

Kupfer C (1962) The projection of the macula in the lateral geniculate nucleus of man. *American Journal of Ophthalmology*, **54**: 597

O'Leary JI, Smith JM, Tidwell M, Harris AB (1965) Synapses in the lateral geniculate nucleus of the primate. *Neurology*, **15**: 548

Saeki N, Fujimoto N, Kubota M, Yamaura A (2003) MR demonstration of partial lesions of the lateral geniculate body and its functional intra-nuclear topography. *Clinical Neurology and Neurosurgery*, **106**: 28

Shacklett DE, O'Connor PS, Dorwart RH, Linn D, Carter JE (1984) Congruous and incongruous sectoral visual field defects with lesions of the lateral geniculate nucleus. *American Journal of Ophthalmology*, **98**: 283

Wada K, Kimura K, Minematsu K, Yamaguchi T. (1999) Incongruous homonymous hemianopic scotoma. *Journal of Neurological Science*, **163**: 179

Further reading

Adler FH, Kaufman PL (eds) (2002) *Adler's Physiology of the Eye. Clinical Application*, 10th edn. St Louis, Mosby

Brouwer B, Zeeman WPC (1925) Experimental anatomical investigation concerning the projection of the retina on the primary optic centres in apes. *Journal of Neurology and Psychiatry*, **6**: 1

Brouwer B, Zeeman WPC (1926) The projection of the retina in the primary optic neuron in monkeys. *Brain* **49**: 1

Chacko LW (1948) Laminar pattern of the lateral geniculate body in the primates. *Journal of Neurology, Neurosurgery and Psychiatry*, **11**: 211

Harrington DO (1946) Automonic nervous system in ocular disease. *American Journal of Ophthalmology*, **29**: 1405

Hickey TL, Guillery RW (1979) Variability of laminar patterns in the human LGN. *Journal of Comparative Neurology*, **183**: 221

Ingvar S (1923) On thalamic evolution: preliminary note. *Acta Medica Scandinavica*, **59**: 696

Kaas JH, Guillery RW, Allman JM (1972) Some principles of organization in the dorsal lateral geniculate nucleus. *Brain and Behaviour Evolution*, **6**: 253

Kanski J (2003) *Clinical Ophthalmology. A Systematic Approach*, 5th edn. London, Butterworth Heinemann

Kanski J (2004) *Clinical Ophthalmology. A Synopsis.* London, Butterworth Heinemann/Elsevier Science

Le Gros Clark WE, Penman GG (1934) The projection of the retina in the lateral geniculate body. *Proceedings of the Royal Society of London*, **114**: 291

Noorden GK von, Middleditch PR (1975) Histological observations in the normal monkey lateral geniculate nucleus. *Investigative Ophthalmology and Visual Science*, **14**: 55

O'Leary JS (1940) A structural analysis of the lateral geniculate nucleus of the cat. *Journal of Comparative Neurology*, 73: 405

Olver J, Cassidy L (2005) *Ophthalmology at a Glance.* Oxford, Blackwell Publishing

Snell RS, Lemp MA (1998) *Clinical Anatomy of the Eye*, 2nd edn. Oxford, Blackwell Publishing

Woollard HM (1926) Notes on the retina and lateral geniculate body in *Tupaia, Tarsius, Nycticebus* and *Hapale. Brain*, 49: 77

Chapter 10

Optic radiations

Anatomy*

Meyer (1907) described the radiations as being divided into three bundles: the superior, inferior and central bundles. The central portion is larger than the superior and inferior portions and contains macular nerve fibres in a wedge arrangement located between the superior and the inferior nerve fibres. The superior nerve fibres originate in the medial aspect of the dorsal nucleus of the lateral geniculate body. The inferior nerve fibres originate from the lateral aspect of the dorsal nucleus of the lateral geniculate body. The superior and central bundles of nerve fibres pass directly posteriorly through the posterior temporal and parietal lobes to their termination in the occipital lobes. The superior fibres remain superior throughout and reach the dorsal lip of the calcarine fissure.

The nerve fibres of the inferior bundle are at first directed anteriorly and laterally superior to and around the inferior horn of the lateral ventricle to form the Flechsig–Archambault–Meyer loop (commonly known as Meyer's loop) (Meyer 1907), after which they turn laterally and posteriorly and proceed through the sublenticular portion of the internal capsule in the temporal lobe until they also reach the visual cortex (Buren & Baldwin 1958). The inferior fibres ultimately reach the ventral lip of the calcarine fissure.

The blood supply to the optic radiations is predominantly from the posterior and middle cerebral arteries. Where the optic radiations pass laterally superior to the inferior horn of the lateral ventricle, the blood supply is by perforating branches of the anterior choroidal artery. Posterior and lateral to the descending horn of the ventricle, the blood supply is from the deep optic branch of the middle cerebral artery. As the optic radiations spread towards the visual cortex, the blood supply is by perforating cortical vessels, predominantly from the calcarine branch of the posterior cerebral artery but also from the middle cerebral artery (Abbie 1938; Francois *et al.* 1958).

---

* This anatomy section is intended as a brief description only. If required, further detail should be sought from appropriate textbooks – see Further reading. The anatomy and pathology sections, in combination, provide a background to the part of the visual pathway covered in this chapter so that the relevant visual field defects can be considered and interpreted appropriately.

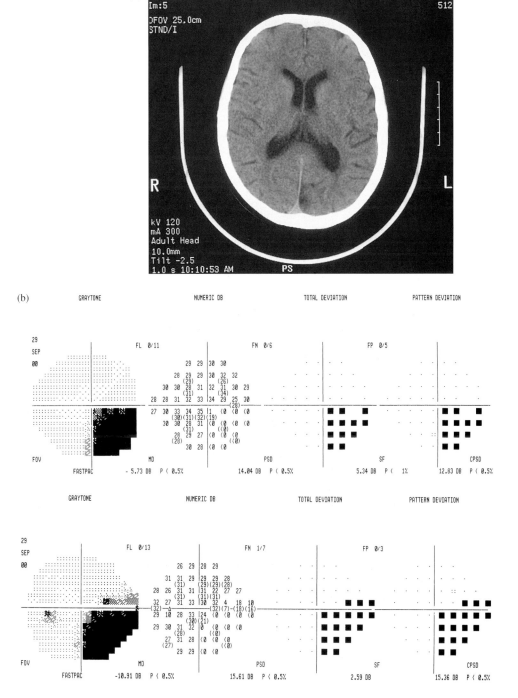

Figure 10.1 Vascular infarct. (a) On neuroimaging there is a low attenuation signal consistent with an infarct. (b) On visual field assessment there is a slightly incongruous right inferior quadrantanopia that does not respect the horizontal meridia.

Pathology*

The optic radiations pass through a large area of the posterior cranial cavity, including the temporal and parietal lobes, before reaching their termination in the occipital lobe. They are therefore susceptible to a number of different types of pathological lesions, including space-occupying lesions and cerebrovascular disorders. Optic radiation lesions are mostly vascular related in either the posterior cerebral artery or middle cerebral artery territories. Vascular disorders include haemorrhage, infarct (Figs 10.1 and 10.2) and arteriovenous malformations (Fig. 10.3). An arteriovenous malformation is a developmental anomalous communication between the arterial and venous systems without intervening capillary beds. Blood is therefore shunted directly from the arteries to the venous circulation, resulting in problems with associated haemorrhage or shunting of blood away from otherwise normal brain tissue.

Space-occupying lesions include primary tumours (Fig. 10.4), secondary metastases and meningiomas (Fig. 10.5). Trauma, infections, demyelination and leukodystrophies are also possible pathologies.

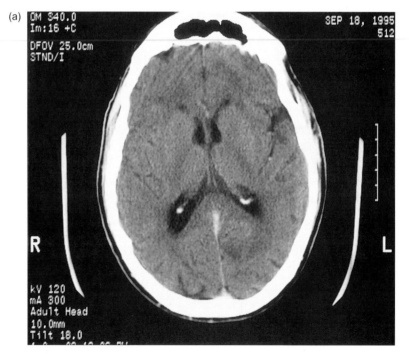

Figure 10.2 Vascular infarct. (a) On neuroimaging there is a left sided low attenuation signal area consistent with an infarct. (b) On visual field assessment there is a right homonymous hemianopia with some involvement of left superior quadrants.

---

* This pathology section is provided as a summary of possible disease processes but by its nature cannot be all inclusive. The reader is directed towards other appropriate textbooks for further detail – see Further reading.

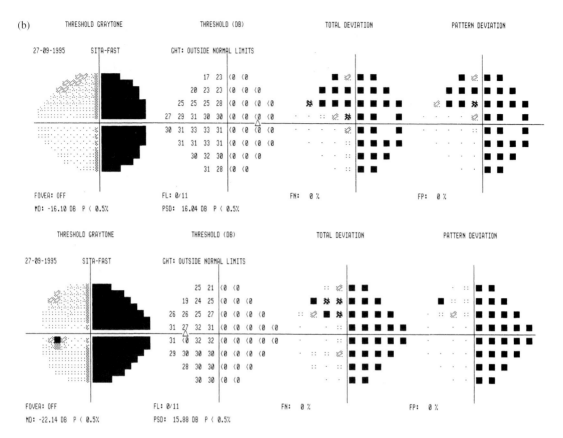

Figure 10.2 (Continued)

The resultant visual deficit and associated signs and symptoms are dependent on the severity and extent of the pathology, as the optic radiations can be involved in their entirety or to a lesser extent by involvement of superior or inferior nerve fibre bundles.

Associated signs and symptoms*

There are frequently other signs of cerebral damage, particularly if the lesion is large. Such signs include eye movement abnormalities, hemiparesis and visual processing abnormalities (Cogan 1960). The temporal lobe lesion can result in complex partial seizures involving abnormal smells, taste, complex visual hallucinations of persons, animals, or known objects. Parietal lobe lesions can result in visual inattention and neglect, aphasia and optokinetic nystagmus abnormality.

---

* This section on associated signs and symptoms is provided so that the practitioner is aware of additional information that can be considered in conjunction with the visual field defect to aid differential diagnosis and localisation of pathology.

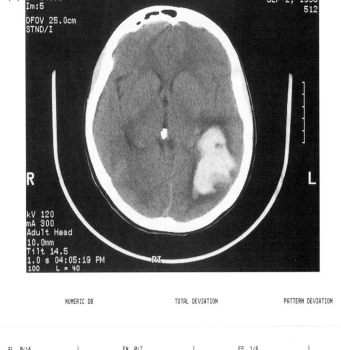

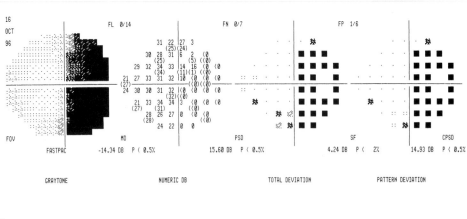

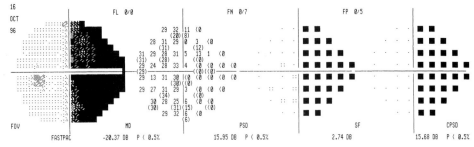

Figure 10.3 Arteriovenous malformation. (a) On neuroimaging a left sided large area of high signal is evident consistent with an arteriovenous malformation. (b) On visual field assessment an incongruous right homonymous hemianopia is documented with macular splitting.

Eye movement abnormalities

Lesions in the parietal lobe involve the descending pathways for saccades and smooth pursuit. Smooth pursuit movements are impaired ipsilaterally (Barton *et al.* 1996) and there is impairment of reflexive saccades. Cogan's sign is a conjugate movement of the eyes to the side opposite the lesion on forced lid closure and this may aid in the diagnosis of the area of lesion. Optokinetic nystagmus will be impaired to the side of the hemianopia and this is a valuable clinical sign in the differential diagnosis of parietal lobe lesions. If the eye movement pathways in the posterior hemispheres are damaged, the optokinetic nystagmus response will be diminished when targets are rotated towards the side of the lesion (away from the hemianopia). There will be a normal large amplitude nystagmus that beats in the direction opposite target movement when targets are rotated towards the intact hemisphere, and will be of diminished amplitude and frequency when targets are rotated towards the damaged hemisphere.

Hemiparesis

The inferior nerve fibres are associated closely to the sensory and motor fibres of the internal capsule. As a result, a lesion in this area may also give rise to a contralateral hemiparesis.

Optic atrophy

Lesions do not generally lead to optic atrophy. This is because the retinal nerve fibres have synapsed in the lateral geniculate body and therefore retrograde degeneration does not occur for the presynaptic nerve fibres prior to the lateral geniculate body. Should optic atrophy be noted, this is usually associated with other pathology such as papilloedema due to raised intracranial pressure.

Pupil abnormalities

Lesions do not generally lead to pupillary defects. Visual field defects will occur with lesions of the optic radiations, but pupillary abnormalities (relative afferent pupillary defect) are not present as these fibres leave the optic tract before reaching the lateral geniculate body to pass to the pretectal nucleus via the superior brachium.

Reading difficulties

Homonymous hemianopias that are apparent on visual field testing can also be reflected in changes of eye movements (Pambakian *et al.* 2000). Leff *et al.* (2001)

stated that the extent of the field defect (particularly right sided visual field loss) had a strong effect on the problems that individual patients experienced during text reading. Patients who had loss of vision within the right parafoveal visual field showed a reduction in the amplitude of eye saccades as well as an increased number of leftward eye movements and an increase in the average number of eye

(a)
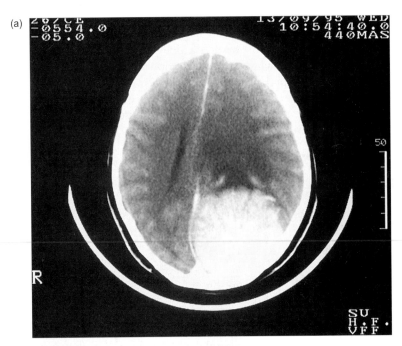

(b)
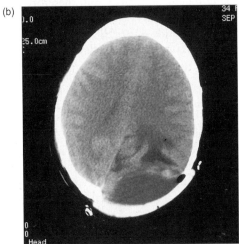

Figure 10.4 Primary space-occupying lesion. On neuroimaging there is a left sided large mass effect in the posterior cranial fossa. Images are shown pre- (a) and postoperatively (b). (c) On visual field assessment there is a right incongruous homonymous hemianopia.

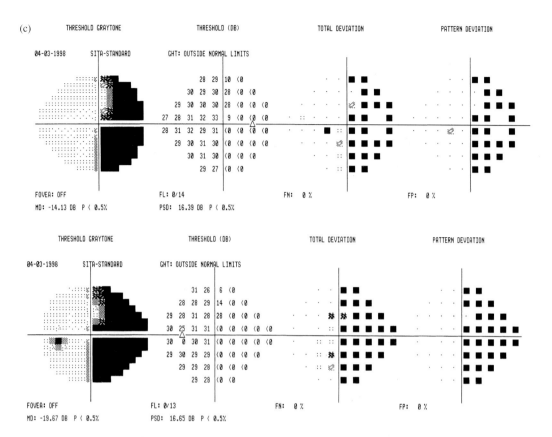

(c)

| THRESHOLD GRAYTONE | THRESHOLD (DB) | TOTAL DEVIATION | PATTERN DEVIATION |

04-03-1998   SITA-STANDARD   GHT: OUTSIDE NORMAL LIMITS

FOVEA: OFF

MD: -14.13 DB   P < 0.5%

FL: 0/14

PSD: 16.39 DB   P < 0.5%

FN: 0 %

FP: 0 %

| THRESHOLD GRAYTONE | THRESHOLD (DB) | TOTAL DEVIATION | PATTERN DEVIATION |

04-03-1998   SITA-STANDARD   GHT: OUTSIDE NORMAL LIMITS

FOVEA: OFF

MD: -19.67 DB   P < 0.5%

FL: 0/13

PSD: 16.65 DB   P < 0.5%

FN: 0 %

FP: 0 %

Figure 10.4 (Continued)

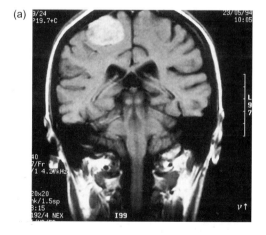

(a)

Figure 10.5 Meningioma. (a) On neuroimaging there is defined mass effect (area of high signal) with downward displacement of neighbouring brain structures. (b) On visual field assessment there is a right superior incongruous quadrantanopia. The right eye also shows inferior nasal visual field impairment due to coexistent glaucoma.

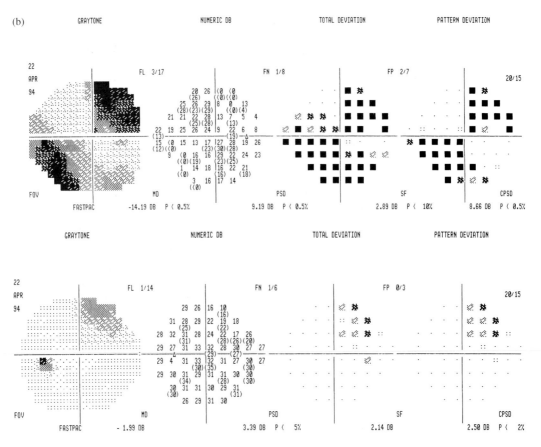

Figure 10.5 (Continued)

movements per word. These results confirm that the right parafoveal field plays an important role in the control of saccades during reading. Patients with left homonymous hemianopia can have difficulty in reading due to problems in leftward scanning movements to return to the beginning of sentences.

Sensory abnormalities

Temporal and parietal lobe lesions can cause higher cortical deficits, including complex partial seizures, auditory or complex visual hallucinations, memory problems or a Wernicke's aphasia (Penfield 1954). Other features of temporal and parietal lobe disease include paroxysmal olfactory or gustatory hallucinations, agraphia, acalculia, graphaesthesia and sensory aphasia. Aphasia is a loss of ability to produce correct speech. Agraphia is impaired writing ability. Acalculia is a form of aphasia characterised by the inability to perform simple mathematical problems. Graphaesthesia is a tactual inability to recognise writing.

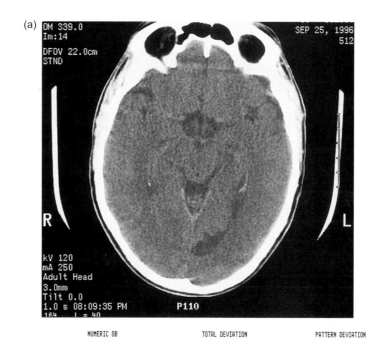

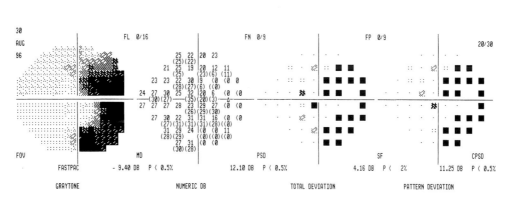

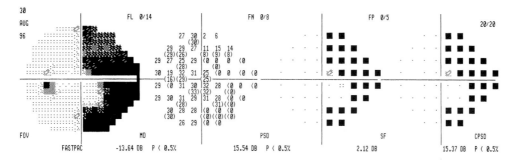

Figure 10.6 Vascular infarct. (a) On neuroimaging there is a left sided area of low attenuation consistent with an infarct. (b) On visual field assessment there is right incongruous homonymous hemianopia.

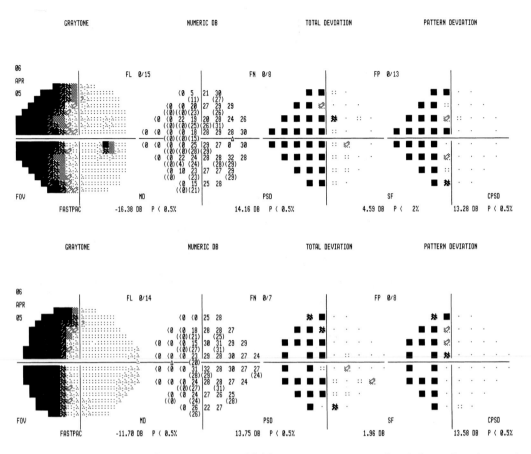

Figure 10.7 Humphrey perimeter visual field assessment: trauma. A right sided cranial involvement has produced a slightly incongruous left homonymous hemianopia.

Visual processing

Defective associate visual processing includes visual agnosia, simultanagnosia, prosopagnosia, complex formed visual hallucinations, alexia, right/left confusion and inability to recognise colours and colour matching (cerebral achromatopsia). These defects result from an interruption of occipital–temporal–parietal projections. Other associated visual processing defects include abnormalities of spatial localisation and motion perception (Mishkin *et al.* 1983) which are produced by an impairment of occipital–parietal pathways.

Agnosia

With agnosia, the patient cannot identify previously familiar objects by sight, despite adequate visual acuity, nor learn to identify new objects by sight alone. When the patient is allowed to feel, smell or listen, the object can be identified.

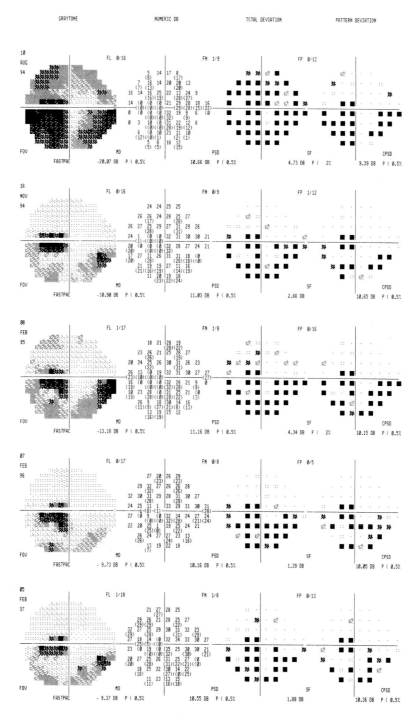

Figure 10.8 Humphrey perimeter visual field assessment: space-occupying lesion. A right sided tumour has produced a left markedly incongruous homonymous hemianopia. There is improvement of visual field function after removal of the tumour with a residual left incongruous quadrantanopia.

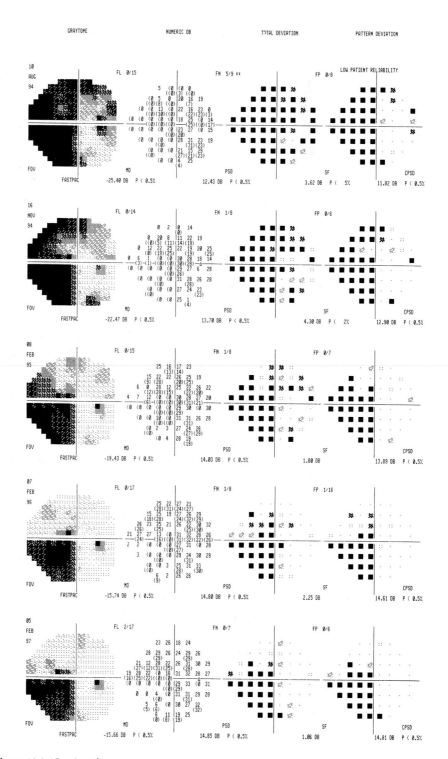

Figure 10.8 (Continued)

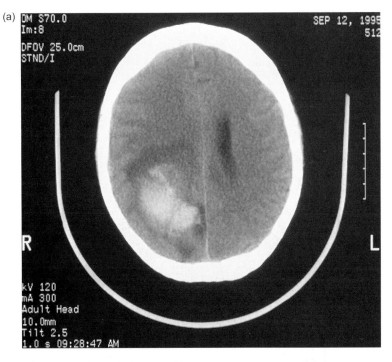

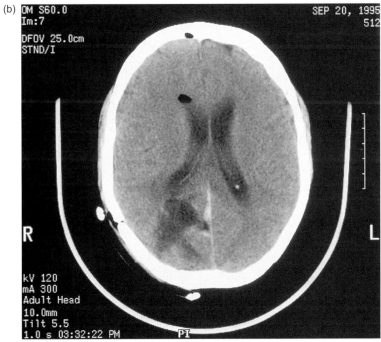

Figure 10.9 Space-occupying lesion. (a,b) On neuroimaging there is a right sided lesion of high signal. Images are shown pre- (a) and postoperatively (b). (c,d) On visual field assessment there is a left incongruous inferior quadrantanopia (c) that is seen to improve postoperatively (d).

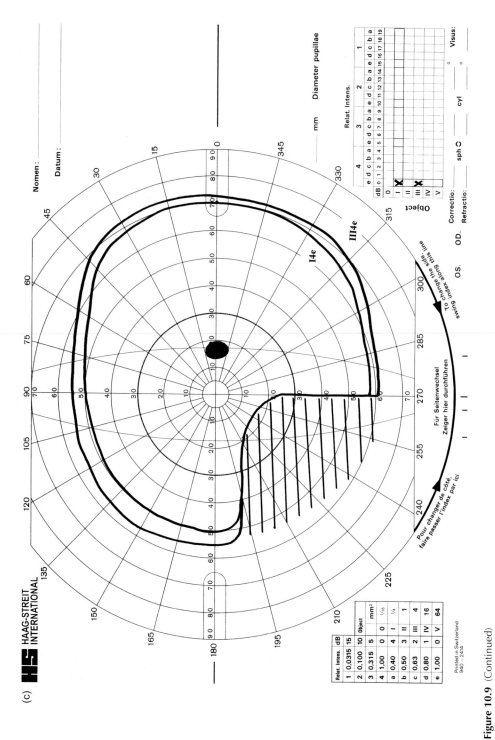

Figure 10.9 (Continued)

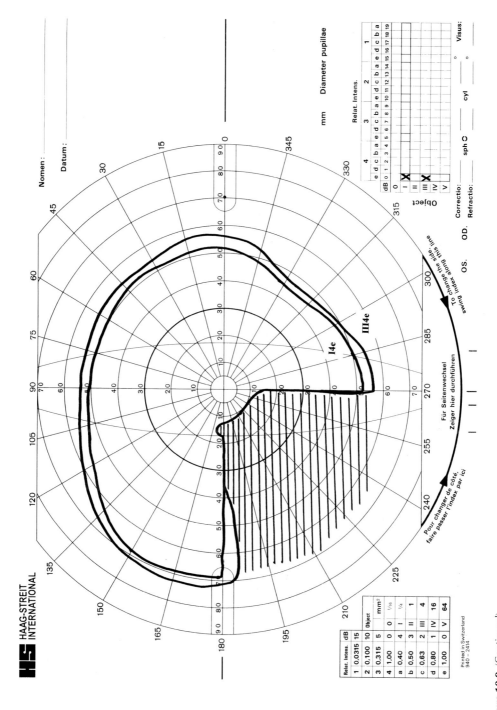

Figure 10.9 (Continued)

(d)

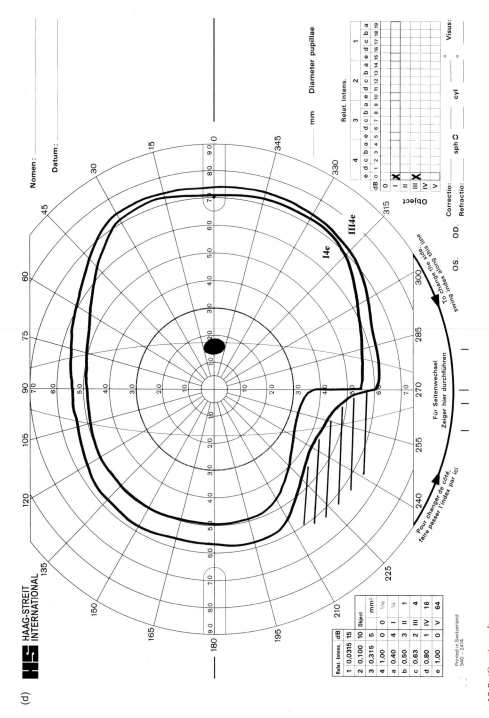

Figure 10.9 (Continued)

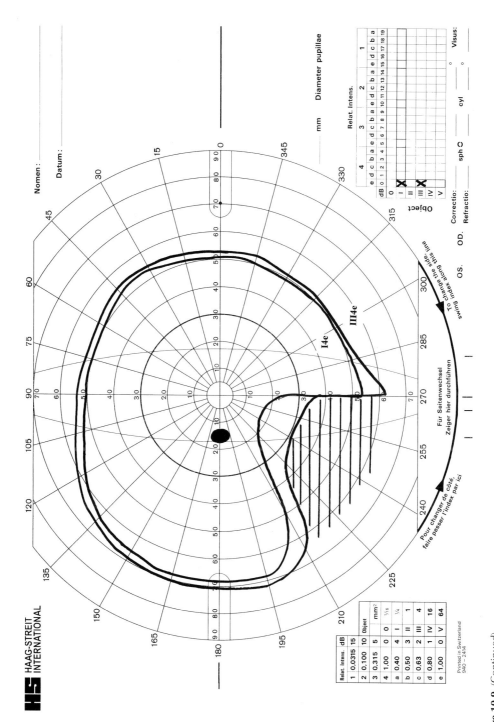

Figure 10.9 (Continued)

Alexia

Alexia is the loss of reading ability in previously literate persons. Pure alexia patients can write. Global alexia includes an inability to read numbers, letters, symbols and words. In less severe alexia, patients can read but with occasional errors and with reduced speed. They use letter-by-letter reading. Almost all lesions are in the left hemisphere, and most are in the medial and inferior occipitotemporal region. Secondary alexia is impaired reading ability due to physical factors, e.g. hemifield slide, unable to read with hemianopic field defect. Bilateral frontal or parietal lesions can impair reading severely due to saccadic dysfunction. Alexia combined with agraphia has been described (Kawahata & Nagata 1988).

Prosopagnosia

With prosopagnosia patients no longer recognise the faces of previously familiar persons, nor learn newly encountered faces (Damasio *et al.* 1982) They use alternative clues to identify people, e.g. non-facial cues such as gait, mannerisms or context in which they met. Lesions are in the medial occipitotemporal cortex and usually bilateral.

Simultanagnosia

Patients are unable to recognise multiple elements in a visual presentation, in that one object or some elements of a scene can be appreciated, but not the scene as a whole.

Visual neglect

Visual neglect is usually left sided with or without hemianopia due to right parietal lobe lesion. Damage to extrastriate regions of the cerebral cortex can lead to hemispatial neglect in which visual stimuli on the contralesion side of space are ignored. Neglect is a multifaceted disorder manifesting itself within different sensory domains and reference frames, and cannot be explained by a simple retinotopic visual deficit. Even when a patient directs their eyes to the left, targets to the left of the body midline are ignored. Neglect can also occur within imagined representations. When patients are asked to describe the features of a square in their home town they may fail to report buildings on its left side. Traditionally, the signs of neglect have been associated with damage to the inferior parietal cortex (Hodgson & Kennard 2000), although recent reports suggest that a temporal locus damage may underlie the phenomenon (Karnath *et al.* 2002).

Halligan *et al.* (1990) reported a significant association between visual field defects and visuospatial neglect. There is debate as to whether visual field defects may exacerbate the behavioural manifestations of neglect. However, the severity of visual neglect may not differ whether with or without visual field deficit.

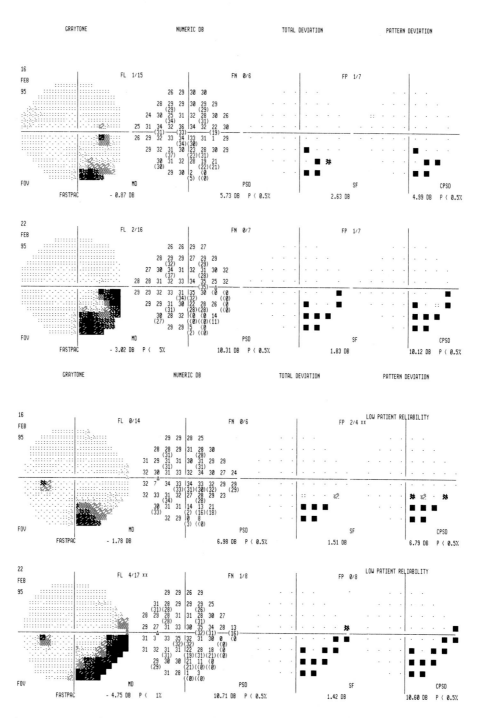

Figure 10.10 Humphrey perimeter visual field assessment: arteriovenous malformation. There is a right slightly incongruous inferior quadrantanopia with progression of the visual field defect over a short period of time due to further haemorrhage of the arteriovenous malformation. The quadrantanopia does not respect the horizontal meridia.

Visual field defects

Visual field defects are dependent on the area involved and the extent of optic radiation inclusion within the lesion. The defects can be hemianopic or quadrantanopic. Lesions of the internal capsule affect the optic radiations while they are still a relatively compact bundle, usually causing a complete homonymous hemianopia. Most often, this defect aligns on the vertical meridian with variable extension toward the horizontal meridian and central vision.

As the optic radiations pass posteriorly towards the striate visual cortex, nerve fibres from corresponding retinal areas lie progressively closer together (Buren & Baldwin 1958). As a result, incomplete hemianopias produced by lesions of the posterior optic radiations are more congruous than those involving the anterior optic radiations. However, a complete hemianopia has no localising value because the extent of incongruity cannot be assessed.

The incongruity, when present, is not as severe as that seen with optic tract and lateral geniculate body lesions, and the more extensive visual field defect in either the left or right field of vision is usually, but not always, in the eye ipsilateral to the lesion (Figs 10.2, 10.4, 10.6 and 10.7).

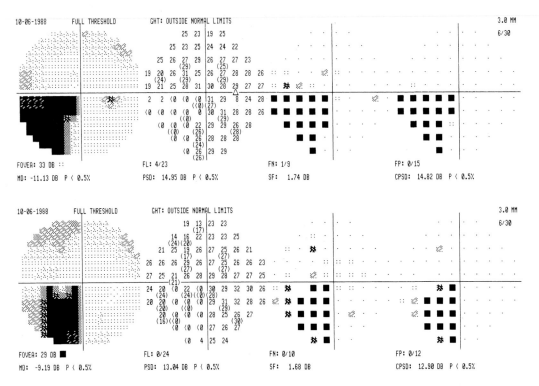

Figure 10.11 Humphrey perimeter visual field assessment: space-occupying lesion. A right sided tumour has produced a left incongruous inferior quadrantanopia which does not align on the horizontal meridia.

Parietal lobe lesion

Homonymous hemianopia affecting primarily the inferior visual fields may be due to involvement of the optic radiations in the superior parietal lobe. Such defects are usually more congruous in appearance than those produced by lesions of the temporal lobe. Since all the optic radiations eventually pass through the parietal lobe, large lesions may produce complete homonymous hemianopia with macular splitting (Figs 10.3 and 10.8). Localised parietal lobe lesions involving the dorsal superior nerve fibres produce an inferior homonymous quadrantanopia and are commonly due to a space-occupying lesion, but may also represent a vascular event (Figs 10.9 and 10.10).

As there is no sharp demarcation of the dorsal fibres from the ventral inferior nerve fibres in this area of the posterior pathway, the visual field defect seldom aligns along the horizontal meridian (Fig. 10.11).

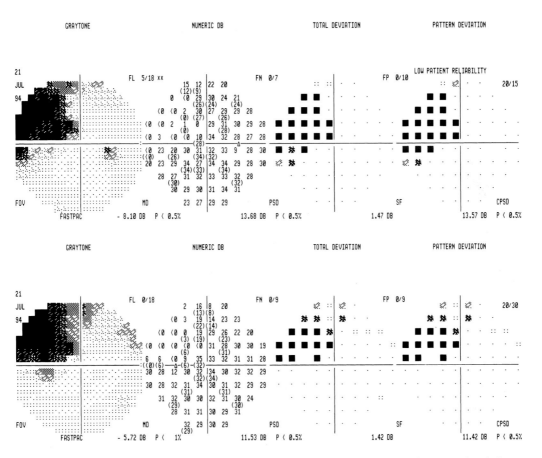

Figure 10.12 Humphrey perimeter visual field assessment: space-occupying lesion. A right sided tumour has produced a left superior quadrantanopia which is slightly incongruous and does not align on the horizontal meridia.

Temporal lobe lesion

A superior homonymous quadrantic defect in the visual fields suggests involvement of either the inferior visual cortex or the inferior optic radiations, and such involvement of the optic radiations may occur in the temporal lobe within Meyer's loop (Marino & Rasmussen 1968) (Figs 10.5 and 10.12). This defect is also commonly termed 'pie in the sky'.

Choice of visual field assessment

Central visual field assessment is usually sufficient to detect most field defects due to pathology of the optic radiations. If pathology is suspected or known but there are no visual field defects centrally, a peripheral visual field test may demonstrate a homonymous loss of visual field in the peripheral field of vision. Peripheral visual field programmes should be undertaken if any doubt exists over the results of a central visual field programme or where full documentation of the entire visual field is required. Careful attention must be paid to the vertical and horizontal meridia.

References

Abbie AA (1938) Blood supply of the visual pathways. *Medical Journal of Australia*, **2**: 199

Barton JJS, Sharpe JA, Raymond JE (1996) Directional defects in pursuit and motion perception in humans with unilateral cerebral lesions. *Brain*, **119**: 1535

Buren JM van, Baldwin M (1958) The architecture of the optic radiations in the temporal lobe of man. *Brain*, **81**: 15

Cogan DG (1960) Hemianopsia and associated symptoms due to parieto-temporal lobe lesions. *American Journal of Ophthalmology*, **50**: 1056

Damasio AR, Damasio H, Hoesen GW van (1982) Prosopagnosia: anatomic basis and behavioral mechanisms. *Neurology*, **32**: 331

Francois J, Neetans A, Collette JM (1958) Vascularisation of primary optic pathways. *British Journal of Ophthalmology*, **42**: 62

Halligan PW, Marshall JC, Wade DT (1990) Do visual field deficits exacerbate visuospatial neglect? *Journal of Neurology Neurosurgery and Psychiatry*, **53**: 487

Hodgson TL, Kennard C (2000) Disorders of higher visual function and hemi-spatial neglect. *Current Opinion in Neurology*, **13**: 7

Karnath HO, Himmelbach M, Rorden C (2002) The subcortical anatomy of human spatial neglect: putamen, caudate nuclei and pulvinar. *Brain*, **125**: 350

Kawahata N, Nagata K (1988) Alexia with agraphia due to the left posterior inferiotemporal lobe lesion: neuropsychological analysis and its pathogenetic mechanisms. *Brain Language*, **33**: 296

Leff AP, Crewes H, Plant GT, Scott SK, Kennard C, Wise RJ (2001) The functional anatomy of single-word reading in patients with hemianopia and pure alexia. *Brain*, **124**: 510

Marino R Jr, Rasmussen T (1968) Visual field changes after temporal lobectomy in man. *Neurology,* **18**: 825

Meyer A (1907) The connections of the occipital lobes and the present status of the cerebral visual affections. *Transactions of the Association of American Physicians*, **22**: 7

Mishkin M, Ungerleider LG, Macko KA (1983) Object vision and spatial vision: two cortical pathways. *Trends in Neuroscience*, **6**: 414

Pambakian AL, Wooding DS, Patel N, Morland AB, Kennard C, Mannan SK (2000) Scanning the visual world: a study of patients with homonymous hemianopia. *Journal of Neurology Neurosurgery and Psychiatry*, **69**: 751

Penfield W (1954) Temporal lobe epilepsy. *British Journal of Surgery*, **41**: 337

Further reading

Adler FH, Kaufman PL (eds) (2002) *Adler's Physiology of the Eye. Clinical Application*, 10th edn. St Louis, Mosby

Barton JJS, Sharpe JA (1997) Smooth pursuit and saccades to moving targets in blind hemifields. A comparison of medial occipital, lateral occipital and optic radiation lesions. *Brain*, **120**: 681

Brain WR (1933) *Diseases of the nervous system*. Oxford, Oxford University Press.

Brouwer B, Zeeman WPC (1925) Experimental anatomical investigation concerning the projection of the retina on the primary-optic centres in apes. *Journal of Neurology and Pscychiatry*, **6**: 1

Geschwind N, Fusillo M (1966) Color-naming defects in association with alexia. *Archives of Neurology*. **15**: 137

Jacobson DM (1997) The localizing value of a quadrantanopia. *Archives of Neurology*, **54**: 401

Kanski J (2003) *Clinical Ophthalmology. A Systematic Approach*, 5th edn. London, Butterworth Heinenmann

Kanski J (2004) *Clinical Ophthalmology. A Synopsis*. London, Butterworth Heinemann/ Elsevier Science

Olver J, Cassidy L (2005) *Ophthalmology at a Glance*. Oxford, Blackwell Publishing

Pallis CA (1955) Impaired identification of faces and places with agnosia for colors. *Journal of Neurology, Neurosurgery and Psychiatry*, **18**: 218

Ranson SW (1943) *The Anatomy of the Nervous System*, Philadelphia, Saunders

Rousseau M, Debrock D, Cabaret M, Steinling M (1994) Visual hallucinations with written words in a case of left parietotemporal lesion. *Journal of Neurology Neurosurgery and Psychiatry*, **57**: 1268

Smith JL (1962) Homonymous hemianopia; a review of 100 cases. *American Journal of Ophthalmology*, **54**: 616

Snell RS, Lemp MA (1998) *Clinical Anatomy of the Eye*, 2nd edn. Oxford, Blackwell Publishing

Spalding JMK (1952) Wounds of the visual pathway: I. The visual radiation. *Journal of Neurology, Neurosurgery and Psychiatry*, **15**: 99

Weinberger LM, Grant FC (1940) Visual hallucinations and their neuro-optical correlates. *Archives of Ophthalmology*, **23**: 166

Chapter 11

Visual cortex

Anatomy*

The nerve fibres of the optic radiations terminate in the visual striate cortex (V1) which is located on the medial aspect of the occipital lobe, superior and inferior to the calcarine fissure. The calcarine fissure has three zones: the posterior macular area, the binocular peripheral area and the anterior monocular peripheral area. The visual cortex is very thin, being only 1.5 mm thick on the floor of the calcarine fissure.

There is a point-to-point localisation of the retina in the visual cortex, each area of the retina being precisely represented in a corresponding area of the visual cortex (Horton & Hoyt 1991; Wong & Sharpe 1999). The superior quadrants of the retinas are represented on the superior lip of the calcarine fissure, and inferior quadrants are on the inferior lip. The central nerve fibres are represented in the extreme tip of the occipital pole, and peripheral nerve fibres are represented by cells lying further forward in the occipital lobe. The most anterior part of the visual cortex represents the extreme nasal periphery of the retina, corresponding to the monocular temporal crescent of the visual fields. The nerve fibres that represent corresponding portions of the fovea of each eye and the immediately surrounding areas occupy a relatively large area in the striate area of the visual cortex of the occipital lobe. There are fewer nerve fibres related to peripheral vision than to central vision. Over half of visual cortex is devoted to the central 10 degrees of nerve fibres; this is termed cortical magnification.

The cortex is supplied predominantly by the posterior cerebral artery and in particular its calcarine branch. A parieto-occipital branch supplies the superior calcarine lip, a posterior temporal branch supplies its inferior lip and a calcarine branch supplies the central region posteriorly. However, there can be marked variation as to which artery supplies the foveal representation in the visual cortex. The middle cerebral artery supplies the posterior aspect of the calcarine sulcus with an anastomosis between posterior and middle cerebral arteries accounting for sparing of the

*This anatomy section is intended as a brief description only. If required, further detail should be sought from appropriate textbooks – see Further reading. The anatomy and pathology sections, in combination, provide a background to the part of the visual pathway covered in this chapter so that the relevant visual field defects can be considered and interpreted appropriately.

macula in cases of posterior cerebral artery occlusion (Abbie 1938; Francois *et al.* 1958; Smith & Richardson 1966).

Pathology*

Pathologies causing unilateral and/or bilateral visual field loss include migraine, trauma, primary and secondary tumours (although the latter are much less common), and vascular abnormalities. Bilateral lesions are not uncommon, since the right and left visual cortices face each other on the medial occipital surface. Lesions can affect both visual cortices either simultaneously or sequentially in vascular pathology (Fig. 11.1), as the right and left posterior cerebral arteries have a common origin from the basilar artery. Trauma and tumours can easily involve both visual cortices as a result of their facing proximity.

Space-occupying lesions

Primary and secondary tumours include infiltrative lesions, glioma and meningioma.

Trauma

In trauma, nerve fibres from the visual pathway can be sheared and avulsion may occur at the lateral geniculate body or visual cortex.

Vascular abnormalities

About 90% of isolated homonymous hemianopias in the absence of other neurological deficits are due to vascular occlusion in the distribution of the posterior cerebral artery (Fig. 11.2). Causes of vascular ischaemia are most frequently cardiac emboli, and vertebrobasilar occlusive disease and arteriovenous malformations. The most common cause, however, is posterior circulation ischaemia. Injury to the vertebral arteries as a result of cervical manipulations is a well documented and dramatic cause of ischaemic syndromes.

Associated signs and symptoms**

Cerebral achromatopsia

Cerebral achromatopsia is a complete loss of colour perception. Lesions are typically in the ventromedial occipital lobe. Bilateral cortical lesions result in

---

*This pathology section is provided as a summary of possible disease processes but by its nature cannot be all inclusive. The reader is directed towards other appropriate textbooks for further detail – see Further reading.

**This section on associated signs and symptoms is provided so that the practitioner is aware of additional information that can be considered in conjunction with the visual field defect to aid differential diagnosis and localisation of pathology.

achromatopsia. The presence of dyschromatopsia indicates some residual colour perception. Unilateral lesions produce colour loss in the contralateral visual hemifield(hemiachromatopsia; Paulson *et al.* 1994) and patients are less aware of colour loss than those with achromatopsia.

Cortical blindness

Cortical blindness is associated with bilateral complete or severe hemianopia with no detectable peripheral visual field. Visual acuity is light perception only or worse. It is distinguished from ocular disease by both normal pupillary light responses and normal fundoscopic examination (Aldrich *et al.* 1987).

Blindness can be divided into permanent and transient forms. The most frequent cause of permanent cortical blindness is cerebrovascular infarction. Transient cortical blindness can occur with metabolic insults, hypertensive encephalopathy, hydrocephalus, trauma and cortical venous thrombosis.

A small minority of patients with cortical blindness behave as though they are not aware of their deficit and insist that they can see (Hartmann *et al.* 1991). This is termed Anton's syndrome. Patients have normal optic disc appearance, pupils, extraocular muscle movement, but no response from the lid reflex in response to light or danger.

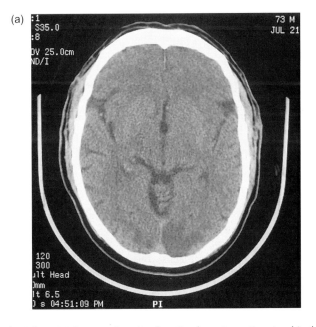

Figure 11.1 Vascular infarct. (a) On neuroimaging there is a low attenuation signal in the occipital lobe greater on the left side than the right. (b) On visual field assessment there is a complete congruous right hemianopia and incomplete left hemianopia (bilateral hemianopia). Central vision is spared – note the decibel values.

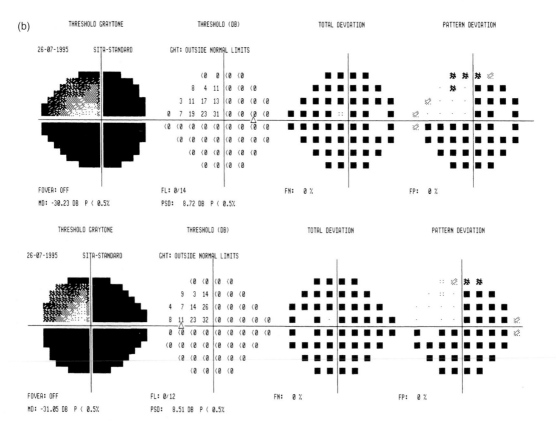

Figure 11.1 (Continued)

Optic atrophy

Optic atrophy is generally absent in patients with visual cortex lesions unless there is other pathology such as papilloedema due to raised intracranial pressure. Presence of optic atrophy generally indicates a lesion of the visual pathway prior to the lateral geniculate body.

Preservation of visual acuity

With preservation of the central field, keyhole vision results with normal visual acuity at distance, but an inability to read large print at near. Despite preservation of normal central vision, such patients behave as though blind, have great difficulty with mobility, and are unable to find large objects close at hand.

Pupil abnormalities

Pupil reactions are typically normal in patients with visual cortex lesions. This is because the pupillary fibres leave the visual pathway prior to the lateral geniculate body and pass to the brainstem nuclei. An afferent pupillary defect is typically seen in visual pathway lesions prior to these pupillary fibres leaving the visual pathway.

Riddoch phenomenon

Certain patients with cortical lesions demonstrate a dissociation of visual perception. In such cases motion is perceived in a portion of visual field that is otherwise blind to static stimuli.

Sensory abnormalities

Visual field defects from visual cortex lesions are often isolated, but can be associated with other signs of higher cortical visual dysfunction such as pure alexia or hemiachromatopsia, whereas visual field defects from lesions located more anteriorly in the visual pathway are usually accompanied by hemiparesis, dysphasia or amnestic problems. Hemiparesis is a paralysis affecting only one side of the body. Dysphasia is a language disorder whereby there is an inability to speak words which one has in mind or to think of correct words, or an inability to understand spoken or written words. Amnestic problems can include a lack or loss of memory or an inability to remember past experiences.

Visual hallucinations

Lesions of the visual cortex may produce formed visual hallucinations. These include paroxysmal scintillating scotomas and light flashes (Anderson & Rizzo 1994).

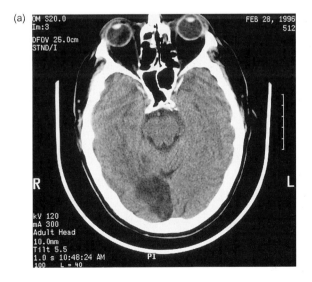

Figure 11.2 Vascular infarct. (a) On neuroimaging there is a low signal at the right occipital lobe. (b) On visual field assessment there is a complete congruous left homonymous hemianopia with macular splitting.

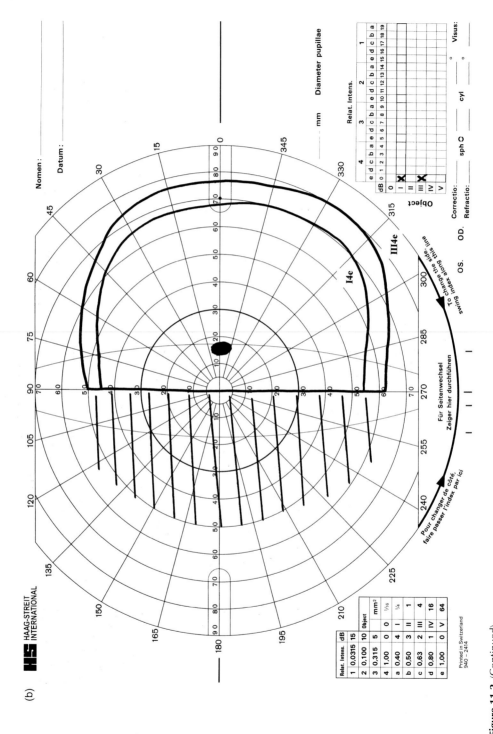

Figure 11.2 (Continued)

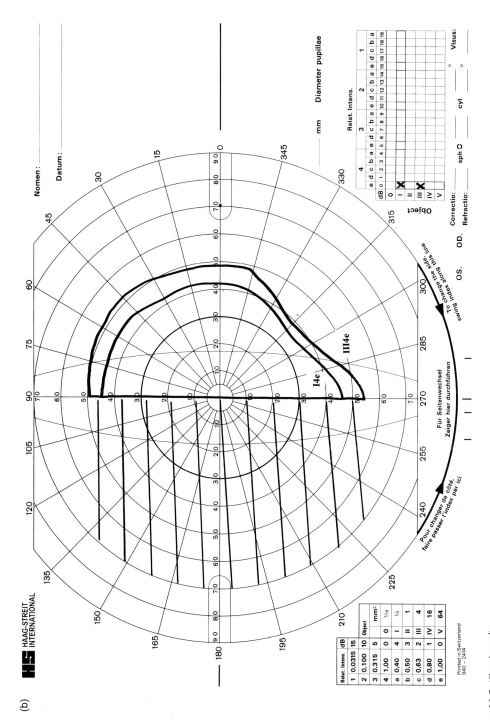

Figure 11.2 (Continued)

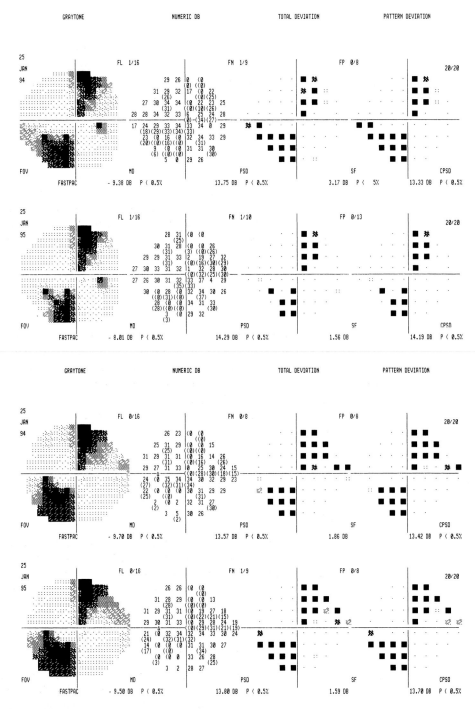

Figure 11.3 Humphrey perimeter visual field assessment: consecutive vascular infarcts. A congruous right superior quadrantanopia and congruous left inferior quadrantanopia are present. The visual field defects occurred due to consecutive infarcts of the occipital lobe. The patient was unaware of the first event, but presented on development of the second inferior quadrantanopia.

Visual field defects

Visual cortex lesions typically produce congruous visual field defects as a result of the direct point-to-point localisation within the visual cortex. There are numerous types of visual field defects that may arise from a visual cortex lesion dependent on the area involved and the extent of the lesion.

Altitudinal visual field defects

Rarely, trauma, tumours or vascular events involving both occipital poles may result in altitudinal field defects. The superior or inferior portions of the visual cortex are damaged. Where the lesion is posterior, the resultant visual field defect may be altitudinal but in a central and scotomatous pattern. Differential diagnosis from altitudinal defects due to ischaemic optic neuropathy can be made by detailed fundus and optic disc examination.

Checkerboard visual field defects

Crossed quadrant hemianopia results when patients develop bilateral quadrantic defects, either simultaneously or consecutively, that involve the superior occipital lobe above the calcarine fissure on one side and on the other side, the inferior occipital lobe below the fissure (Felix 1926). Such defects have also been termed checkerboard fields and occur infrequently (Fig. 11.3).

The upper and lower calcarine lips can be involved separately by ischaemia because the lips have separate blood supplies.

Homonymous hemianopia

Bilateral homonymous hemianopia

Large bilateral occipital lobe lesions produce bilateral complete hemianopic visual field defects resulting in cortical blindness. Bilateral incomplete hemianopia (Fig. 11.1) can be distinguished from bilateral optic nerve or ocular disease by the high congruity of the visual field defects and step defects along the vertical meridian which indicate the hemifield nature of the visual loss.

Unilateral homonymous hemianopia

Focal destruction of the visual cortex will produce a homonymous contralateral hemifield defect, often with macular sparing. Defects are highly congruous, with virtually identical defects in the two eyes. An isolated congruous homonymous hemianopia in the absence of other neurological signs is most commonly caused by an occipital lobe infarct from an occlusion in the posterior cerebral artery territory.

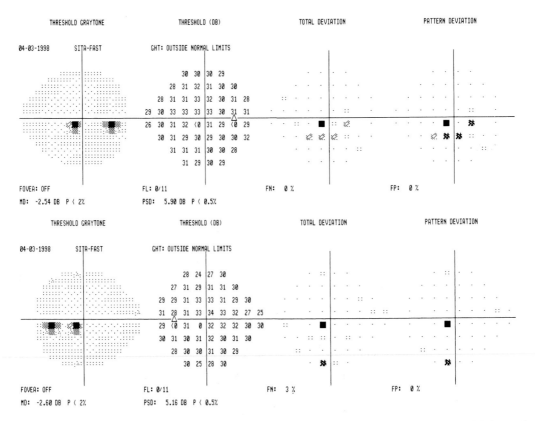

Figure 11.4 Humphrey perimeter visual field assessment: vascular infarct. A congenital left macular hemianopia scotoma is documented – note the decibel values and probability plots.

Complete destruction of the visual cortex will cause complete visual loss in the contralateral visual hemifield with macular splitting (Fig. 11.2).

Macular involvement

Macular hemianopia

Occipital lobe lesions located more posteriorly in the visual cortex may produce primarily central field defects that can break out into the periphery. Damage to the tip of the occipital cortex, as might occur from a head injury, will give rise to congruous homonymous macular defects (Fig. 11.4). Congruity remains a feature of such visual field defects.

Macular sparing

Occlusion of the posterior cerebral artery can produce a macular sparing congruous homonymous hemianopia. If macular sparing occurs, it is diagnostic of an occipital

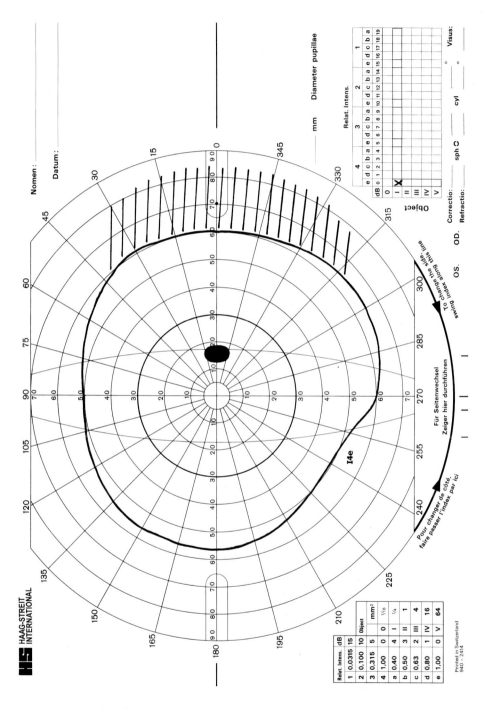

Figure 11.5 Goldmann perimeter visual field assessment: temporal crescent loss. The visual field results appear normal apart from loss of the temporal crescent from 60 degrees peripherally.

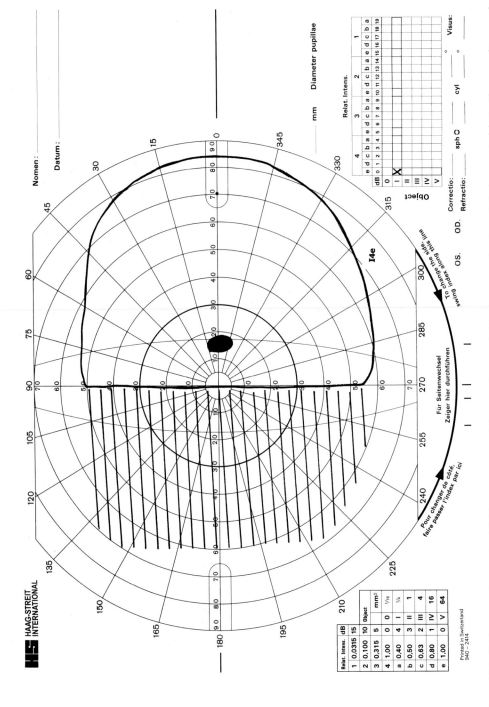

Figure 11.6 Goldmann perimeter visual field assessment: spared temporal crescent. A homonymous hemianopia is documented, but with a spared temporal crescent on the affected side from 60 degrees peripherally.

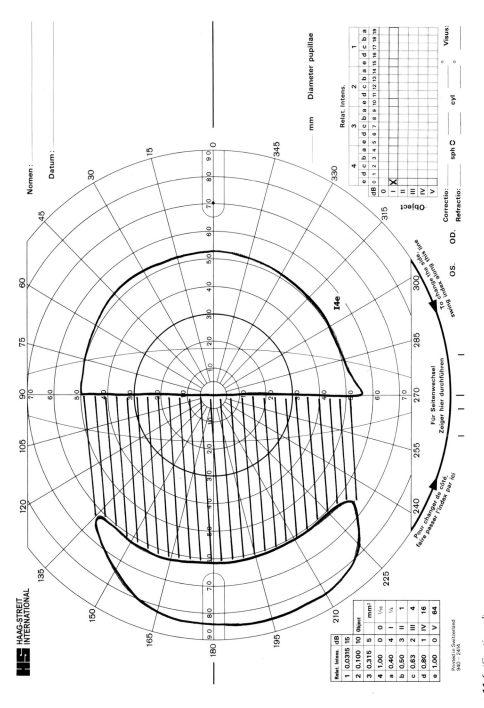

Figure 11.6 (Continued)

lobe lesion, since it is rarely encountered with lesions outside the visual cortex and is therefore of localising value. Macular sparing occurs due to the separate blood supply of the posterior cerebral artery and middle cerebral artery to the visual cortex (Smith & Richardson 1966; Ehlers 1975). The macular fibres typically receive vascular supply at the occipital cortex from the middle cerebral artery.

If homonymous hemianopias include the foveal region as well as peripheral vision, this is called macula-splitting homonymous hemianopia (Fig. 11.2). This can occur in posterior cerebral artery ischaemia in patients whose entire visual cortex is supplied by that artery. It may also occur, however, with complete lesions of the optic tract, lateral geniculate body and optic radiations; therefore other signs should be sought to aid differential diagnosis.

Scotomas

The degree of localisation at all levels of the cortex entails that even small lesions may produce sharply outlined scotomas in corresponding locations in both visual fields. A lesion of the occipital pole alone causes homonymous central hemianopia scotomas (Fig. 11.4). This can occur with watershed infarcts during systemic hypoperfusion.

Slightly more anterior lesions in the middle zone of the visual cortex may cause homonymous peripheral scotomas. The highly congruent, homonymous nature of these defects and their restriction to one hemifield differentiate these from ocular causes of central or paracentral scotomas.

Bilateral occipital lobe lesions produce bilateral homonymous scotomas. Occasionally, such scotomas have some degree of central sparing such that a ring scotoma is produced.

Temporal crescent defect or sparing

Unilateral lesions of the anterior occipital lobe involving the unpaired peripheral nasal nerve fibres will produce a monocular defect in the extreme temporal visual field. This visual field defect is crescentic in shape and its widest extent is along the horizontal meridian where it extends from 60 degrees out to approximately 90 degrees (Fig. 11.5). Because of its particular shape, a defect in this region has been termed a temporal crescent or half moon syndrome. A near complete lesion that spares only the most anterior portion of the visual cortex causes a hemianopia with sparing of the temporal crescent. This sparing of the outer temporal field in the eye to the side of the hemianopia is a feature of localised occipital lobe infarct. The hemianopia involves the whole nasal hemifield of the ipsilateral eye, but the temporal hemifield of the contralateral eye spares a crescent shaped island of vision in the far periphery (Fig. 11.6) (Benton *et al.* 1980).

Choice of visual field assessment

Central visual field assessment is usually sufficient to detect most field defects due to pathology of the striate visual cortex. If pathology is suspected or known but there are no visual field defects centrally, a peripheral visual field test may demonstrate a loss of temporal crescent. Equally, where there is suspected sparing of the temporal visual field it is advisable to choose a peripheral visual field assessment to explore this area. Peripheral visual field programmes should be undertaken if any doubt exists over the results of a central visual field programme or where full documentation of the entire visual field is required. Careful attention must be paid to the vertical meridian and central fixation.

References

Abbie AA (1938) Blood supply of the visual pathways. *Medical Journal of Australia*, **2**: 199

Aldrich MS, Alessi AG, Beck RW, Gilman S (1987) Cortical blindness: etiology, diagnosis and prognosis. *Annals of Neurology*, **21**: 149

Anderson SW, Rizzo M (1994) Hallucinations following occipital lobe damage: the pathological activation of visual representations. *Journal of Clinical and Experimental Neurology*, **16**: 651

Benton S, Levy I, Swash M (1980) Vision in the temporal crescent in occipital infarction. *Brain*, **103**: 83

Ehlers N (1975) Quadrant sparing of the macula. *Acta Ophthalmologica*, **53**: 393

Felix CH (1926) Crossed quadrant hemianopsia. *British Journal of Ophthalmology*, **10**: 191

Francois J, Neetans A, Collette JM (1958) Vascularisation of primary optic pathways. *British Journal of Ophthalmology*, **42**: 62

Hartmann JA, Wolz WA, Roeltgen DP, Loverso FL (1991) Denial of visual perception. *Brain Cognition*, **16**: 29

Horton JC, Hoyt WF (1991) The representation of the visual field in human striate cortex. A revision of the classic Holmes map. *Archives of Ophthalmology*, **109**: 816

Paulson HL, Galetta SL, Grossman M, Alavi A (1994) Hemiachromatopsia of unilateral occipitotemporal infarcts. *American Journal of Ophthalmology*, **118**: 518

Smith CG, Richardson WFG (1966) The course and distribution of the arteries supplying the visual (striate) cortex. *American Journal of Ophthalmology*, **61**: 1391

Wong AMF, Sharpe JA (1999) Representation of the visual field in the human occipital cortex. A magnetic resonance imaging and perimetric correlation. *Archives of Ophthalmology*, **117**: 208

Further reading

Adler FH, Kaufman PL (eds) (2002) *Adler's Physiology of the Eye. Clinical Application*, 10th edn. St Louis, Mosby

Barton JJS, Sharpe JA (1997) Smooth pursuit and saccades to moving targets in blind hemifields. A comparison of medial occipital, lateral occipital and optic radiation lesions. *Brain*, **120**: 681

Clark WEL (1942) The visual centers of the brain and their connections. *Physiology Review*, **22**: 205

Duvernoy HM, Delon S, Vannson JL (1981) Cortical blood vessels of the human brain. *Brain Research*, **7**: 519

Harrington DO (1961) Character of the visual field in lesions of the temporal and occipital lobe. *Archives of Ophthalmology*, **66**: 778

Holmes G (1931) A contribution to the cortical representation of vision. *Brain*, **54**: 470

Kanski J (2003) *Clinical Ophthalmology. A Systematic Approach*, 5th edn. London, Butterworth Heinemann

Kanski J (2004) *Clinical Ophthalmology. A Synopsis*. London, Butterworth Heinemann/ Elsevier Science

Kupersmith MJ, Vargas ME, Yashar A, Madrid M, Nelson K, Seton A, Berenstein A (1996) Occipital arteriovenous malformations: visual disturbances and presentation. *Neurology*, **46**: 953

Olver J, Cassidy L (2005) *Ophthalmology at a Glance*. Oxford, Blackwell Publishing

Pallis CA (1955) Impaired identification of faces and places with agnosia for colors. *Journal of Neurology, Neurosurgery and Psychiatry*, **18**: 218

Snell RS, Lemp MA (1998) *Clinical Anatomy of the Eye*, 2nd edn. Oxford, Blackwell Publishing

Spalding JMK (1952) Wounds of the visual pathway: Part II. The striate cortex. *Journal of Neurology, Neurosurgery and Psychiatry*, **15**: 169

Stensaas MA, Eddington DK, Dobelle WH (1974) The topography and variability of the primary visual cortex in man. *Journal of Neurosurgery*, **40**: 747

Troost BT, Newton TH (1975) Occipital lobe arteriovenous malformations. *Archives of Ophthalmology*, **93**: 250

Weinberger LM, Grant FC (1940) Visual hallucinations and their neuro-optical correlates. *Archives of Ophthalmology*, **23**: 166

Chapter 12

Differential diagnosis

Standard brain studies by magnetic resonance imaging or computerised tomography scans may provide too few sections of orbital or basal skull structures. Visual field analysis can help to identify the likely area of visual pathway involved and provide precise instructions to the radiologist as to the specific areas to be imaged.

Lesions in certain areas of the visual pathway may produce associated signs and symptoms specific to that site of lesion, e.g. post fixational blindness in optic chiasm lesions. Please refer to each section of the visual pathway for further descriptions of signs and symptoms.

Age

Some conditions predilect for older age groups, such as cerebrovascular accidents (stroke). Certain space-occupying lesions also have age predilections, such as craniopharyngioma in children and young adults.

Congruity

Congruity is the extent of symmetry of the visual field defect in either eye, and can only be assessed by direct comparison of the visual field results from either eye. The presence of a complete congruous homonymous hemianopia does not distinguish between a lesion of the optic tract, lateral geniculate body, optic radiations or visual striate cortex.

Incomplete incongruous hemianopia indicates an optic tract lesion, lateral geniculate body lesion or lesion of the optic radiations. The closer the lesion is to the optic chiasm the greater the incongruity of visual field defects. Conversely, congruity of visual field defects will increase towards the visual cortex.

Therefore, if a homonymous hemianopia is grossly incongruous, a lesion of the optic tract should be suspected. As the optic tract leaves the posterior aspect of the optic chiasm, homonymous hemifield nerve fibres from each eye are not yet paired, so incomplete optic tract lesions typically produce incongruous homonymous hemianopias. Incongruous wedge shaped visual field defects suggest lesions of the lateral geniculate body, particularly if central fixation is involved, although these lesions are rare.

The optic radiations fan laterally and inferiorly from the lateral geniculate body, sweeping around the anterior aspect of the lateral ventricles. The optic radiations are the most vulnerable part of the visual pathway. The most antero nerve fibres form Meyer's loop which contains the inferior nerve fibres. A lesion of the temporal lobe involving this loop of optic radiations produces a superior quadrantic hemianopia or quadrantanopia. If such a visual field defect is documented and is incongruous, it suggests a temporal lobe lesion. If the superior quadrantanopia is perfectly congruous, it could be due to either a lesion of the temporal lobe or of the visual cortex.

Although parietal lobe lesions can produce an inferior quadrantanopia, in practice many lesions involving the parietal lobes cause complete homonymous hemianopia which is indistinguishable from hemianopias due to visual cortex lesions.

Eye movement generation

Assessment of optokinetic nystagmus may be useful in determining the cause of an isolated homonymous hemianopia that has no other associated neurological deficits (Heide *et al.* 1996; Ghika *et al.* 1998; Heide & Kompf 1998). If the eye movement pathways in the posterior hemispheres are damaged, the optokinetic nystagmus response will be diminished when targets are rotated towards the side of the lesion (away from the hemianopia). There will be a normal large amplitude nystagmus that beats in the direction opposite target movement when targets are rotated toward the intact hemisphere; nystagmus will be of diminished amplitude and frequency when targets are rotated towards the damaged hemisphere. This is called a positive optokinetic nystagmus sign.

In most cases, the combination of a homonymous hemianopia and optokinetic nystagmus asymmetry is characteristic of a parietal lobe lesion which is often a space-occupying lesion. Rarely, occipital lobe lesions may also cause optokinetic nystagmus asymmetry.

There is impaired smooth pursuit movement to the side of the lesion; ipsilateral horizontal smooth pursuit difficulties in unilateral cortical lesions can result in replacement of smooth pursuit movements by a series of saccadic movements (cogwheel movements) (Leigh & Tusa 1985; Bogousslavsky & Regli 1986; Lekwuwa & Barnes 1996). Impaired saccadic movement occurs to the contralateral side of lesion (Steiner & Melamed 1984).

Fundus and anterior segment abnormalities

Presence of fundus and optic disc pathology will indicate anterior visual pathway disease rather than retrochiasmal pathology. Papilloedema may be noted due to raised intracranial pressure which can cause visual field defects in addition to those caused by the primary intracranial pathology. Ocular media pathology will be detected by slit lamp examination.

Ocular motility abnormalities

Associated cranial nerve palsy can indicate the site of lesion dependent on the type and multitude of cranial nerves involved. Cranial nerve palsy may be particularly noted with lesions in the optic chiasm area. Other ocular motor abnormalities particularly associated with lesions involving the optic chiasm include hemifield slide phenomenon, post-fixational blindness and see-saw nystagmus (Rowe 1996). Conjugate deviation of the eyes (Cogan's sign) (Steiner & Melamed 1984) and third cranial nerve palsy are also seen with temporal lobe lesions.

Optic atrophy

Retinal nerve fibres synapse in the lateral geniculate body. Lesions involving the presynaptic nerve fibres may result in optic atrophy due to retrograde degeneration of retinal nerve fibres. This atrophy may be band shaped, as with bow tie atrophy in optic chiasm lesions. Optic atrophy is uncommon with lesions involving post-synaptic nerve fibres in the optic radiations and visual cortex, unless there is associated secondary papilloedema which will directly affect the nerve fibres at the optic disc.

Pupil abnormalities

An afferent pupillary conduction defect is suggestive of a lesion prior to the lateral geniculate body, as the visual pathway up to the optic tracts contains retinal nerve fibres that subserve both visual and pupillomotor functions.

Sensory abnormalities

Patients may complain of ocular pain in conditions such as glaucoma or retrobulbar neuritis. Pain will also be a symptom in cases of migraine.

Conditions such as pituitary adenoma or craniopharyngioma will be associated with general signs related to hormone dysfunction such as Cushing syndrome, acromegaly, obesity and diabetes insipidus.

If a hemianopia is accompanied by hemiplegia or hemianaesthesia, the lesion is typically in the posterior part of the internal capsule.

A temporal lobe lesion can result in complex partial seizures involving abnormal smells and taste. Abnormalities of smell may also occur with tumours (e.g. meningioma) arising from the olfactory groove. Parietal lobe lesions can result in aphasia.

Type of visual field defect

Certain types of visual field defect are more associated with specific parts of the visual pathway (Fig. 12.1).

An altitudinal visual field defect involves two quadrants of either the superior or inferior visual field and is typically seen in optic neuropathies. It may rarely be due to bilateral symmetric involvement at a higher level, including bilateral lesions affecting the medial aspects of the lateral geniculate body and bilateral occipital lobe lesions.

Arcuate visual field defect is caused by selective damage to the superior or inferior retinal nerve fibre bundles and is typical of optic disc disease.

Hemianopia is a complete defect involving one-half of the visual field. A heteronymous hemianopia involves opposite sides of the visual field (e.g. lesions of the optic chiasm typically produce bitemporal heteronymous hemianopias). A homonymous hemianopia involves the same side of the visual field in each eye (e.g. lesions

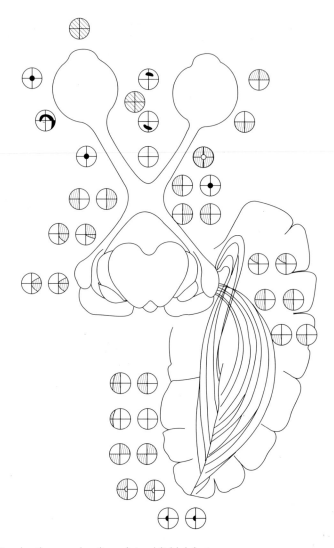

Figure 12.1 Visual pathway and outline of visual field defects.

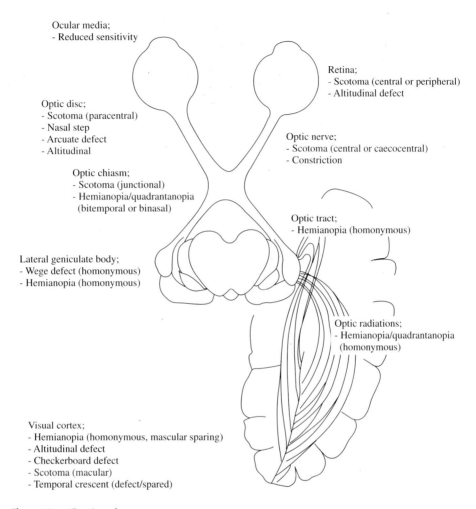

Ocular media;
- Reduced sensitivity

Retina;
- Scotoma (central or peripheral)
- Altitudinal defect

Optic disc;
- Scotoma (paracentral)
- Nasal step
- Arcuate defect
- Altitudinal

Optic nerve;
- Scotoma (central or caecocentral)
- Constriction

Optic chiasm;
- Scotoma (junctional)
- Hemianopia/quadrantanopia
  (bitemporal or binasal)

Optic tract;
- Hemianopia (homonymous)

Lateral geniculate body;
- Wege defect (homonymous)
- Hemianopia (homonymous)

Optic radiations;
- Hemianopia/quadrantanopia
  (homonymous)

Visual cortex;
- Hemianopia (homonymous, mascular sparing)
- Altitudinal defect
- Checkerboard defect
- Scotoma (macular)
- Temporal crescent (defect/spared)

Figure 12.1 (Continued)

of the retrochiasmal pathways typically produce homonymous hemianopias). The presence of macular splitting or macular sparing homonymous hemianopias can aid differential diagnosis between visual cortex lesions and lesions located more anteriorly in the visual pathway.

Quadrantanopia is a complete defect involving a quadrant of each visual field. Heteronymous quadrantanopia involves opposite sides of the visual field and either superior or inferior quadrants. Homonymous quadrantanopias involve the same side of the visual field in each eye and either superior or inferior quadrants. These may be produced by temporal, parietal or occipital lobe lesions.

Scotomas are absolute or relative areas of depressed visual function surrounded by normal vision, which may be central, paracentral or caecocentral in type. These are commonly seen in retinal, optic disc and optic nerve disease, although macular hemianopic scotomas may be seen in occipital lobe lesions. Homonymous scotomas are indicative of visual cortex lesions, rather than retinal or optic nerve lesions, because of their congruity and homonymous nature.

Sector-shaped visual field defects start as small scotomas on the temporal side of the visual field and end as complete sectorial loss. These are commonly associated with optic disc disease. Sector-shaped defects that are homonymous and involve central fixation indicate a lesion of the lateral geniculate body.

Table 12.1 outlines unilateral versus bilateral visual field loss and potential location within the visual pathway.

Visual acuity

Symptoms of central vision involvement with homonymous hemianopia indicate a more anterior visual pathway lesion. Central and caecocentral scotomas in optic nerve disease will impair visual acuity. Macular splitting hemianopia does not generally disrupt central visual acuity completely. Table 12.2 outlines the possible diagnoses associated with retained visual acuity in constricted visual fields.

Visual field defect progression

Progressive versus sudden visual field loss can aid diagnosis of pathology. Homonymous visual field defects typically develop slowly if they are due to the presence of

Table 12.1 Pathway location and visual field loss.

Unilateral visual field loss	Generally prior to the optic chiasm – optic nerve and retina
Bilateral visual field loss	Asymmetric visual field defects with different patterns are usually retinal, optic nerve and optic disc Symmetric visual field defects are usually optic chiasm or post optic chiasm lesions (optic tract, lateral geniculate body, optic radiations and visual cortex)

Table 12.2 Constricted visual field with retained central visual acuity.

Possible diagnoses
Late glaucoma
Retinitis pigmentosa
Post-papilloedema optic atrophy
Drusen of the disc
Bilateral occipital infarcts with macular sparing
Malingering

Table 12.3 Differential diagnosis of glaucoma.[a]

Glaucoma versus...	
Retina	Pathology identified on fundus examination Retinal visual field defects relate to the specific area of pathology, e.g. scotoma where a toxoplasmosis infection exists Generally there is no specific pattern of visual field loss Glaucoma has specific visual field types such as paracentral scotomas that develop into arcuate defects and nasal steps with progression to generalised constriction of the visual field
Optic disc and optic nerve	Differential diagnosis can be difficult as this is the site of pathology for glaucoma also Detailed examination of the optic disc is required. Look for cupping of the optic disc in glaucoma and any identifiable features of other pathology such as a congenital abnormality (optic disc pit, tilted disc, hypoplasia) or acquired abnormality (ischaemic optic neuropathy, papilloedema) Drusen of the optic disc should be excluded and may require ultrasound of the optic disc if buried within the tissue Intraocular pressure will be elevated in many cases of glaucoma but not in normal tension types
Optic chiasm	Patients can have optic nerve compression dependent on the anatomy of the optic chiasm and location of the pathology The general visual field defect is that of a heteronymous hemianopia or quadrantanopia, but patients can also have nasal visual field involvement and scotomas; however, the latter are usually central in type rather than paracentral Other signs and symptoms related to optic chiasm involvement should be sought such as Cushing syndrome, acromegaly, hemifield slide phenomenon
Optic tract, lateral geniculate body and optic radiations	The usual visual field defect is that of homonymous hemianopia or quadrantanopia with varying extent of congruity Associated signs and symptoms can help localise the area of pathology such as presence of hemiparesis, hormone dysfunction, alexia, agnosia, visual neglect, achromatopsia, and lack of optic atrophy and relative afferent pupillary defect (pathology post lateral geniculate body) Central fixation is always involved with a lateral geniculate body pathology, but is usually spared until very late in the course of glaucomatous pathology
Visual cortex	Visual field defects are typically bilateral and highly congruous; this is highly unusual in glaucoma Scotomas, if present in visual cortex pathology, are of a homonymous and congruous nature and are typically not paracentral in nature There are no fundus signs with visual cortex lesions unless there is coexistent pathology; pupillary function is normal

[a]It must be remembered that glaucoma can coexist with intracranial pathology, e.g. Fig. 10.5.

Table 12.4 Pathway location and associated signs and symptoms.

Location	Signs and symptoms
Retina	Fundus appearance: pathology is visible with ophthalmoscopy Visual field defects are monocular Visual field defects are seen in relation to their position from the fovea Visual field defects can cross both the horizontal and vertical meridia Abnormal visual acuity and colour with macula or fovea involvement
Optic nerve	Fundus appearance: optic disc pallor, optic disc swelling Visual field defects are monocular Visual field defects point towards the disc as nerve fibres travel towards the disc Scotomas can enlarge and merge into an arcuate visual field defect Optic disc changes are seen by ophthalmoscopy Reduced visual acuity, contrast sensitivity and colour vision with afferent pupillary defect
Optic chiasm	Bow tie atrophy, see-saw nystagmus, diplopia, strabismus Bitemporal hemianopia visual field defect is most common Visual field defects respect the vertical meridian in early loss of visual function Pituitary adenoma is the most common pathology and visual field defects start superiorly and progress inferiorly Extensive visual field defect is associated with reduced colour vision, visual acuity and afferent pupillary defect Associated signs and symptoms include diabetes insipidus, obesity, Cushing syndrome, acromegaly, postfixational blindness and hemifield slide phenomenon
Optic tract	All visual field defects are homonymous and respect the vertical meridian Macular fixation is split but there is potential for normal central visual acuity Relative afferent pupillary defect Incongruous visual field defects are typical Associated signs and symptoms include hemiparesis, hormone dysfunction and optic atrophy
Lateral geniculate body	Homonymous hemianopia visual field defect is typical Incongruous visual field defects Visual field defects point to and include fixation There is potential for normal central visual acuity Associated signs include optic atrophy but normal pupillary function
Optic radiations	Temporal lobe lesions result in a more dense superior visual field defect Parietal lobe lesions result in a more dense inferior visual field defect Incongruous visual field defects are typical There is potential for normal central visual acuity No relative afferent pupillary defect Associated signs and symptoms include agnosia, aphasia, alexia, achromatopsia, acalculia, hallucinations, hemiparesis, optokinetic abnormality and visual neglect
Visual cortex	Visual field defects can respect the horizontal meridian Congruous visual field defects Temporal crescent visual field defects are asymptomatic There is potential for normal central visual acuity Macular sparing in hemianopic visual field defects Macular hemianopia visual field defects Associated signs and symptoms include Anton's syndrome, achromatopsia, alexia, hallucinations and Riddoch phenomenon

intracranial tumour and develop rapidly when they are due to vascular abnormalities such as haemorrhage, emboli, thrombosis or infarction.

In many cases of homonymous hemianopia due to intracranial tumour, there is progression of the visual field defects from the periphery to the centre. When the intracranial tumour is removed and compression of the visual nerve fibres removed, improvement first occurs in the central visual fields and continues toward the periphery.

Visual perception

Retinal disease may be associated with the appreciation of flashes and floaters, such as with retinal detachment. Optic nerve disease is associated with reduction in visual acuity, colour vision and contrast sensitivity. A relative afferent pupillary defect may also be noted. Patients may complain of amaurosis fugax or transient visual obscurations. A temporal lobe lesion can result in complex visual hallucinations of persons, animals or known objects. Parietal lobe lesions can result in visual inattention and neglect, and optokinetic nystagmus abnormality.

Monocular diplopia associated with homonymous hemianopia indicates a visual cortex lesion. Visual hallucinations involving light flashes indicate a visual cortex lesion. Formed hallucinations indicate temporal and parietal lobe lesions. Other symptoms associated with visual cortex lesions include Riddoch phenomenon and cortical blindness.

Tables 12.3 and 12.4 are intended as further aids to diagnosis and localisation of pathology site.

References

Bogousslavsky J, Regli F (1986) Pursuit eye defects in acute and chronic unilateral parieto-occipital lesions. *European Neurology*, **25**: 10

Ghika J, Ghika-Schmid F, Bogousslavsky J (1998) Parietal motor syndrome: a clinical description in 32 patients in the acute phase of pure parietal strokes studied prospectively. *Clinical Neurology and Neurosurgery*, **100**: 271

Heide W, Kompf D (1998) Combined deficits of saccades and visuo-spatial orientation after cortical lesions. *Experimental Brain Research*, **123**: 164

Heide W, Kurzidim K, Kompf D (1996) Deficits of smooth pursuit eye movements after frontal and parietal lesions. *Brain*, **119**: 1951

Leigh RJ, Tusa RJ (1985) Disturbances of smooth pursuit caused by infarction of occipito-parietal cortex. *Annals of Neurology*, **17**: 185

Lekwuwa GU, Barnes GR (1996) Cerebral control of eye movements. I The relationship between cerebral lesion sites and smooth pursuit deficits. *Brain*, **119**: 473

Rowe FJ (1996) Visual disturbances in chiasmal lesions. *British Orthoptic Journal*, **53**: 1

Steiner I, Melamed E (1984) Conjugate eye deviation after acute hemispheric stroke: delayed recovery after previous contralateral frontal lobe damage. *Annals of Neurology*, **16**: 509

Chapter 13

Visual field artefacts and errors of interpretation

Inaccurate visual field results can be documented for a variety of reasons, and ensuing errors of interpretation can have serious consequences for the diagnosis and ultimately the management decisions for the individual patient.

Artefacts of visual field results may relate to the instructions given to the patient, the set-up of the patient at the instrument, or the patient's ability to perform the visual field assessment.

Poor instruction can give rise to incorrect patient responses to the stimuli presented. Poor set-up and failure to maintain correct set-up throughout the test can result in lens rims defects and ptosis artefacts. Poor patient ability to perform visual field assessment can relate to learning curve, fatigue, and lack of understanding producing fixation losses and false answers.

There are a number of external variables that must be considered with regard to the visual field result. These include anatomical features of the face (e.g. prominent brow or nose), interference with ocular media and perception of stimuli (e.g. ptosis, miotic pupil, uncorrected refractive error, cataract), attention and age of the patient, and technique of the examiner (explanation of the test and patient set-up) (Haas *et al.* 1986; Johnson *et al.* 1989).

Esterman programme assessment

The Humphrey field analyser owner's manual states that distance glasses should be worn if the patient needs them to function normally. In general, however, distance glasses should not be worn, as the frames may obscure part of the peripheral field, thus producing an artefact in the visual field (Steel *et al.* 1996). This is particularly important as many modern frames are small aperture and could easily produce an artefact in the visual field by blocking stimuli presented more peripherally in the perimeter bowl.

The stimulus intensity is 10 decibels which is sufficiently bright to obtain a response without need of a spectacle correction. However, where there is a marked refractive error and doubt is expressed at the visual field result, the visual field test may be repeated using the spectacle correction and a comparison of responses obtained.

Fatigue

Where a patient suffers fatigue during visual field assessment, sensitivity of the visual field decreases during the examination. This becomes more pronounced as the examination time increases; it is greater when the second eye is examined and it increases with the age of the patient (Wild *et al.* 1991; Hudson *et al.* 1994). Therefore, the greater the increase in mean deviation, the older the patient (Gonzalez de la Rosa & Pareja 1997). Use of a faster test strategy may be required if fatigue or patient illness is likely to impede performance, e.g. fastpac as opposed to a full threshold programme (Nordmann *et al.* 1994; O'Brien *et al.* 1994). The patient may be given rest periods during the test and may control the rest periods themselves by keeping the response button pressed down continuously during Humphrey visual field assessment (this has the effect of pausing the machine).

Hysterical visual loss and malingering

Hysteria is a neurosis; patients may complain of an inability to see small detail or read, or perhaps a marked visual field defect. These symptoms are real to the patient. The malingering patient deliberately pretends to have visual loss.

Hysteria or malingering should be suspected if the defect does not match a presumed diagnosis or if the defect is not physiologically possible, e.g. a large visual field is plotted with a small target compared to a smaller visual field plotted with a larger target (Fig. 13.1). All pathology must be ruled out before making the diagnosis of functional visual loss.

Typical visual field defects documented in these patients include hemianopia (Keane 1977), constricted visual field and spiral defects (Fig. 13.2) (Smith & Baker 1987). Where reduced visual acuity is also reported stereoacuity tests, such as TNO or Frisby stereotests, may be used to aid diagnosis as bilateral good visual acuity is required to achieve a good level of stereoacuity.

Learning curve

When undergoing measurement of visual fields, a number of patients experience a learning curve (Anderson 1992). Most patients learn perimetry quickly during the first visual field assessment after the first few stimulus points have been presented, and as a result the first test is often accurate. Some patients, however, do not provide an accurate visual field result until the second test. For this reason, a demonstration test may be run before the first test (Rowe 1998). The learning curve involves learning to respond consistently during the test; with experience, patients are noted to respond to more dim stimuli and to stimuli presented further away from the central fixation point (Werner *et al.* 1988; Autzen & Work 1990). Therefore, the usual artefact from an initial test is an overall reduction in sensitivity of the visual field.

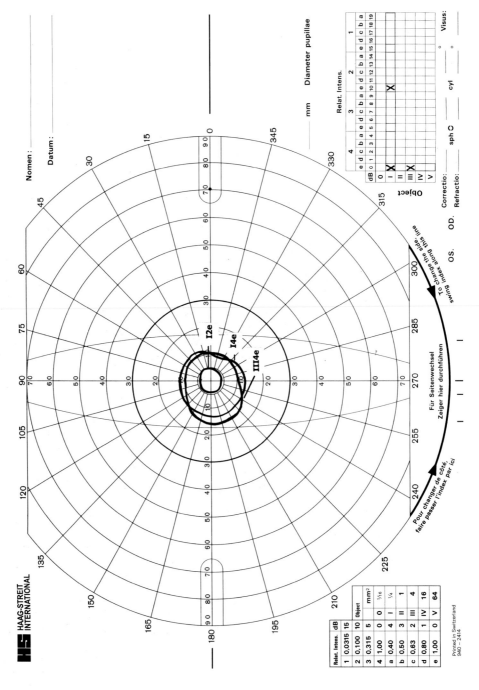

Figure 13.1 Goldmann perimeter visual field assessment: functional defect. The visual field is constricted with more constriction for a larger target size compared to a smaller target size and with crossover of isopters.

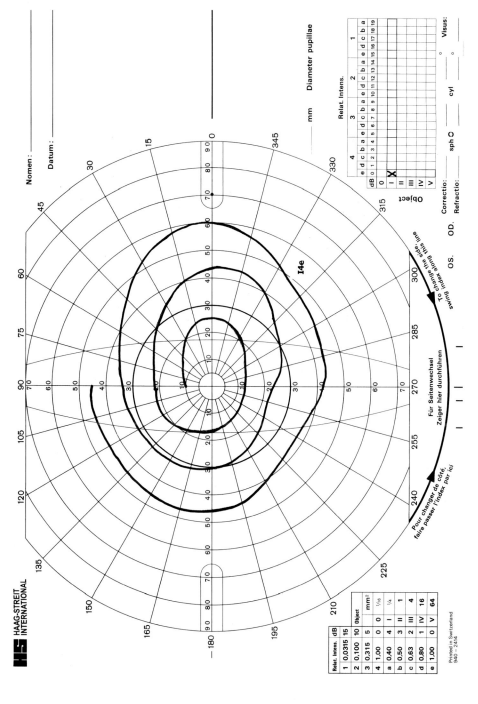

Figure 13.2 Goldmann perimeter visual field assessment: functional defect. There is a spiral visual field effect.

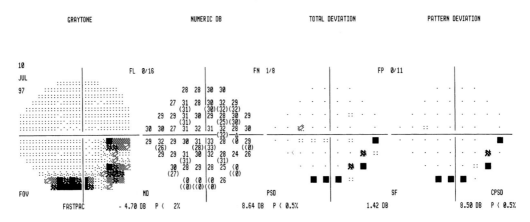

Figure 13.3 Humphrey perimeter visual field assessment: lens rim defect. There is an inferior lens rim defect in the right eye involving outer edge points. Note the decibel values of <0 despite the presence of neighbouring points at 25–29 decibels.

Localised visual field defects which are typically seen relating to papilloedema and optic nerve head pathology are therefore unlikely to be artefacts (see Figs 10.1 and 11.2). Probability plots will often allow detection of localised visual field loss despite over-riding reduction in sensitivity.

Where suspicion exists regarding the reliability of the first test, the patient may be recalled for a second test at a later stage, and the second test taken as the baseline if felt to be more accurate. Thorough explanation of the test prior to running the programme and questioning of the patient as to their understanding of the test will help in obtaining a reliable result.

Lens rim defects

Poorly positioned lenses will interfere with visual perception, as stimuli will not be seen by the patient if blocked by a poorly positioned lens (Zalta 1989; Henson & Earlam 1995; Donahue 1998). Visual field defects are usually located between 25 and 30 degrees if related to a lens artefact (Zalta 1989). Where possible, it is advisable to use the patient's own single lens prescription unless these are small frames. Otherwise, wide aperture lenses should be used with the eye positioned as close to the lens as possible. A give-away as to the presence of a lens rim defect is the sudden drop of sensitivity at the tested point to less than 0 decibels where neighbouring points closer in to fixation have not shown such a drop in sensitivity (Figs 13.3 and 13.4). Visual field defects extend over the horizontal and/or vertical meridia.

Observer interpretation

When interpreting the printout of results, it may be tempting to interpret the greyscale only as this provides an immediate view of the visual field. However,

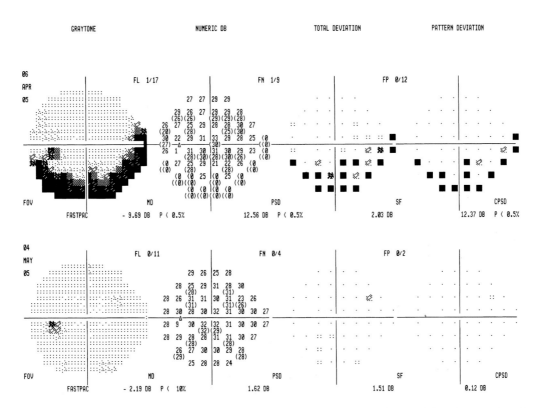

Figure 13.4 Humphrey perimeter visual field assessment: lens rim defect. The left eye has an inferior lens rim defect involving outer edge points predominantly and extending from the nasal visual field around to the blind spot. Note the <0 decibel values. On subsequent assessment with correct lens position there is a normal visual field result.

by interpreting the greyscale only, some areas of localised loss in the visual field may not be noted where there is diffuse visual loss also, and further progression of an existing visual field defect may not be noted. A true indication of the extent of loss is not therefore obtained. Occasionally, interpretation of the greyscale only resulting in false diagnosis of progressive visual field loss has related to the use of a new printer ribbon/cartridge where the quality of the greyscale print is darker with the new cartridge, but the probability plots clearly indicate the same extent of visual loss (Rowe 1998).

Ocular variables

Age gradually depresses the visual field. Light-difference sensitivity decreases with age partly due to age-related loss of nerve fibres (Balazsi *et al.* 1984) and increased condensation of the media (see Fig. 1.2 for variability in normal visual field boundaries in varying ages).

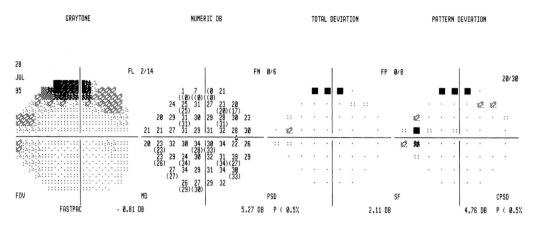

GRAYTONE　　　　　NUMERIC DB　　　　　TOTAL DEVIATION　　　　　PATTERN DEVIATION

28
JUL
95

FL 2/14　　　　　　　FN 0/6　　　　　　FP 0/8　　　　　　　20/30

```
          1   7  (0  21
        ((0)((0)((0)
     24  25  31  27  23  20
        (25)        (20)(17)
  20 29  31  30  29  28  30  23
        (31)        (31)
  21 21 27  31  29  31  32  28  30
  20 23 32  30  34  30  34  22  26
     (23)    (28)(33)
     23 29  34  30  32  31  39  29
     (26)    (34)    (34)(27)
        27  34  29  31  34  30
        (27)            (33)
        26  27  29  32
        (29)(30)
```

FOV

FASTPAC

MD
- 0.81 DB

PSD
5.27 DB P < 0.5%

SF
2.11 DB

CPSD
4.76 DB P < 0.5%

Figure 13.5 Humphrey perimeter visual field assessment: ptosis. A visual field defect appears in the right superior field. Note the <0 decibel values.

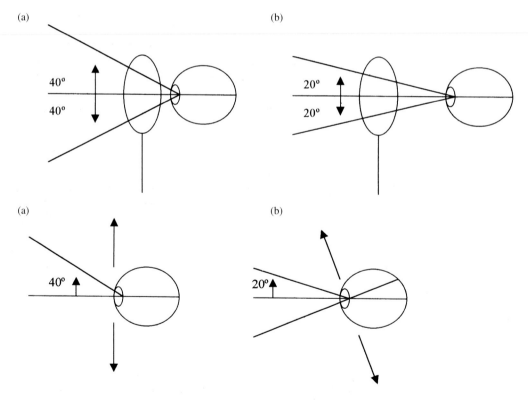

Figure 13.6 Head position representation (a) Correct head position with wide field of view. (b) Incorrect position due to the head being tilted, producing a restricted field of view and resulting in a lens rim defect.

Miosis depresses the visual field and can exaggerate the size and depth of existing visual field defects. Pupil diameter less than 2 mm produces visual field loss as pupil constriction dims both the intensity of the stimulus and the intensity of the background. This is a problem when assessing patients requiring miotics for glaucoma (Mikelberg *et al.* 1987; Lindermuth *et al.* 1989; Webster *et al.* 1993; Edgar *et al.* 1999).

Abnormalities that interfere with media clarity reduce illumination and therefore depress the visual field; they also exaggerate existing visual field defects (Spaeth 1980; Guthauser *et al.* 1987; Guthauser & Flammer 1988). See Chapter 4 for visual field assessment results in the presence of cataract.

The presence of ptosis or a tendency for the lid to droop during testing may produce a superior artefact of the visual field (Meyer *et al.* 1993; Klingele *et al.* 1995; Federici *et al.* 1999) (Fig. 13.5) and the lid should be taped open to prevent this. Ptosis produces an artefact with sudden reduction in sensitivity from normal values to 0 decibels in the superior field of vision (Cahill *et al.* 1987). This may appear in both eyes if bilateral or just one eye, or the second eye tested if fatigue related.

Patient instruction and set-up

The correct set-up and instructions that should be given to the patient have been outlined in Chapter 2 for both Humphrey and Goldmann visual field assessment. In essence, the patient should be seated comfortably holding the response button in either hand and instructed to look straight ahead at the central light. Their head should be placed squarely in the chin rest and against the forehead rest. Where trial frame lenses are used, these are placed before the tested eye as close to the eye as possible without touching the eyelashes.

When mapping the peripheral boundaries of the visual field using Goldmann perimetry, the patient is instructed to press the response button as soon as they are aware of a white light moving into their field of vision. When assessing static points in Humphrey and Goldmann visual field assessment, the patient is instructed to press the response button any time they are aware of a brief flash of white light, one at a time, outside central fixation during the test, some bright and some dim.

It is important to monitor the patient continually throughout the test, to give encouragement and reassurance, and to ensure the continued correct set-up for the duration of the test.

Patient positioning

Correct positioning of the patient at the machine is necessary to ensure the patient's head is upright and not tilted to the side or backwards (Fig. 13.6). This is particularly important where patients do not wear full frame spectacles and a reading correction is required as an additional lens. The additional lens should be positioned as close to the patient's eye as possible with the visual axis located through the centre of

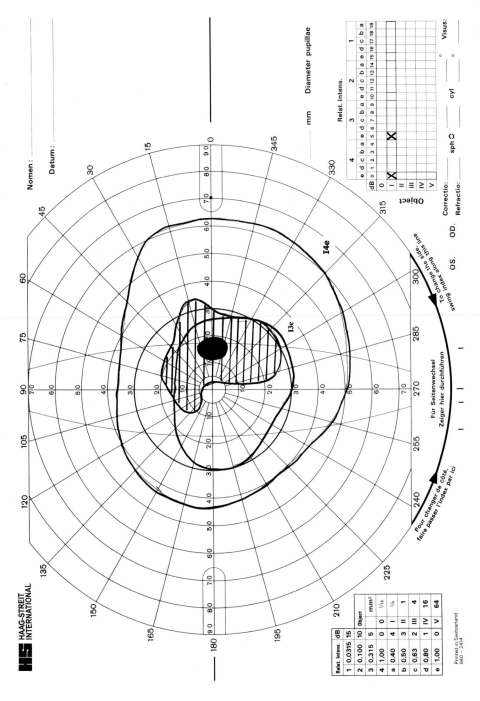

Figure 13.7 Goldmann perimeter visual field assessment: refractive scotoma. Note the extensive enlargement of the blind spot. This reduces considerably when the blind spot is assessed using the appropriate refractive correction for the central visual field.

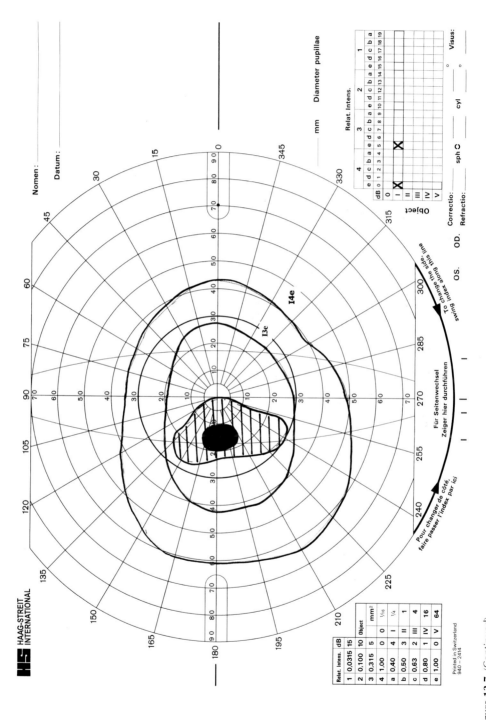

Figure 13.7 (Continued)

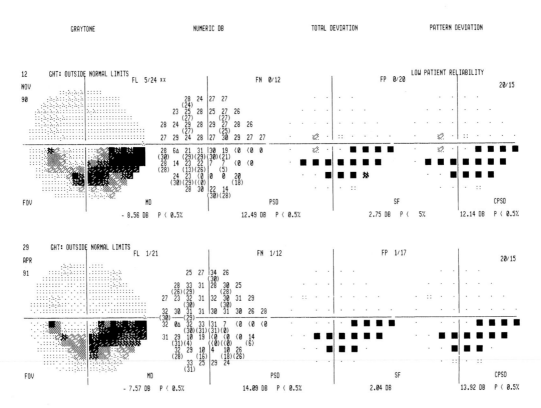

Figure 13.8 Humphrey perimeter visual field assessment: fixation losses. Fixation losses are evident on the first visual field assessment, but there are no false positive or false negative scores. Probability plots show definite visual field loss. On repeated assessment there is good reliability and a similar pattern of visual field loss is evident.

the lens. Poorly positioned lenses will interfere with visual perception by the patient, resulting in a lens rim defect.

Performance difficulties

Artefacts related to the patient's ability to perform visual field assessment may be due to poor understanding of the test, slow reflexes, concentration failure, positioning problems with lens edge rim defects, and artefacts from lid position, most notably ptosis.

Good instructions can alleviate many of these problems as will allowance of rest time plus encouragement and reassurance during the test.

Refractive errors

Uncorrected or inappropriately corrected refractive errors can lead to enlarged blind spots on visual field assessment, and constriction of visual field, particularly

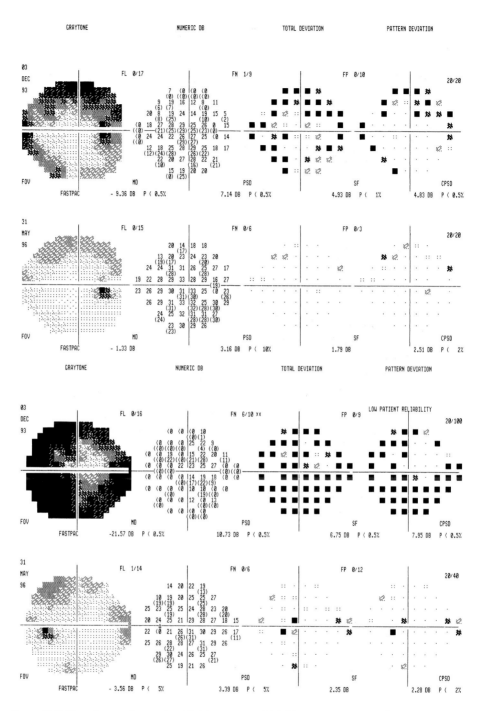

Figure 13.9 Humphrey perimeter visual field assessment: high false negative score. In this case with papilloedema, the right eye shows superior arcuate visual field loss with some inferior nasal field involvement. There is good reliability of assessment in this eye. The left eye shows inferior arcuate visual field loss with development of superior arcuate deficit also. There is a high false negative score, but the visual field loss is still quite evident and the false negative score is probably related to the extent of visual field impairment.

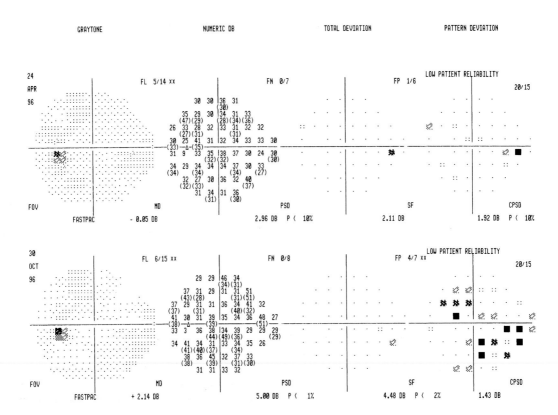

Figure 13.10 Humphrey perimeter visual field assessment: high false positive score (normal visual field). This left eye result does not specifically show a high false positive score in the first result but is increased in the second result. There are fixation losses and the visual field results are recorded as low patient reliability. Note the decibel values; these range up to 47 decibels in the first assessment and up to 51 decibels in the second assessment. The corrected pattern standard deviation shows affected points in relation to these values.

the central visual field function. Refractive errors, if uncorrected, can also result in enlargement of other visual field defects. Defocus effectively enlarges the stimulus size, but will reduce the luminance (Atchison 1987; Henson & Morris 1993; Weinreb & Perlman 1986). These visual field errors can be eliminated with the correct prescription (Fig. 13.7); refractive errors greater than 1 dioptre should be corrected and the prescription given according to the patient's age and instrument optics. Incorrect spectacle corrections can also cause artefacts due to reduced light sensitivity which may produce local or generalised visual field loss. It is therefore important to ensure reading corrections are worn when assessing the central visual field in particular.

A reading correction should be worn during central visual field assessment, and a cylinder prescription should be given where the prescription is ≥1.00 dioptre. Suggested sphere additions are shown in Table 13.1 for Goldmann perimetry. The Humphrey perimeter will calculate the desired prescription on the basis of a distance prescription and the given age of the patient.

Table 13.1 Correction of refractive error[a].

Age (years)	Addition (DS)
30–40	+1.00
40–45	+1.50
45–50	+2.00
50–55	+2.50
55–60	+3.00
>60	+3.25

[a]If dilated at any age, use an addition of +3.25 DS.

Reliability indices

The purpose of reliability indices is to indicate the reliability of the visual field result. However, such indices may on occasion be misleading in relation to fixation loss and false negative scores. Fixation instability may certainly occur with poor fixation, but in addition, fixation instability may occur because of an ill-defined blind spot, presence of nystagmus or head movement during the test. These factors can be accounted for and, in fact, the visual field result is often reliable in many of these instances, particularly if the patient has been visually observed in addition to the catch trials (Fig. 13.8).

Some reliability problems may relate to false negative responses. Throughout the test, a stimulus is projected at a level above threshold at a point which has already had a positive response to a certain decibel value. The patient should therefore respond to this; however, if there is no response, this is recorded as a false negative. Repeated high false negative responses have been found in patients already with visual field defects rather than normals, providing further evidence that false negative responses are more indicative of true defects than of poor patient reliability (Katz *et al.* 1991). High false negative scores may be seen in patients with early onset of visual loss, as there may be relative scotomas with varying visual responses in this area (Fig. 13.9). Visual field results are usually reliable. High false negative scores may also be a sign of fatigue and allowing the patient a break during the test may alleviate this problem.

During the test, the projection device is at times moved, or clicks without presenting a stimulus. Should the patient respond despite the absence of a stimulus, this is recorded as a false positive. A high false positive score is often seen in 'trigger happy' patients who press the response button frequently despite not seeing stimuli. These patients also continue to respond to actual stimuli, with the result that stimuli are presented at consecutively higher sensitivities (Figs 13.10 and 13.11). This will continue beyond the upper limit of 51 decibels if the patient continues to press the response button. The mean deviation value shifts well into the positive area, producing artificial defects in the pattern deviation. Abnormally high sensitivity decibel values are thus achieved and visual field results are therefore unreliable.

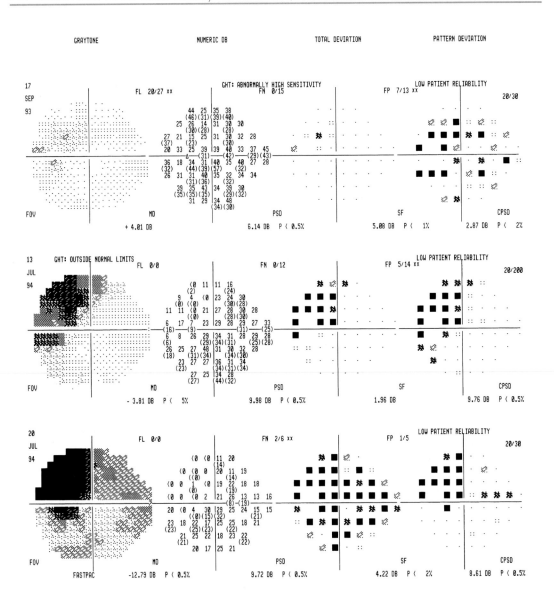

Figure 13.11 Humphrey perimeter visual field assessment: high false positive score (abnormal visual field). This is a case with pituitary adenoma. The results for either eye show high fixation loss and false positive scores with decibel values ranging up to 60. The corrected pattern standard deviation shows affected points in relation to these values. It is not possible to determine true visual field loss from these results. On further assessment there is improvement in reliability with more appropriate decibel values for the age of patient and it is possible to determine the extent of bitemporal visual field loss.

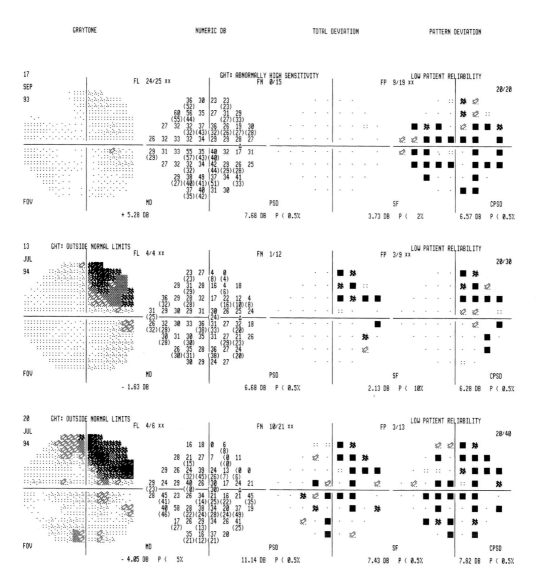

Figure 13.11 (Continued)

References

Anderson DR (1992) *Automated Static Perimetry*. St Louis, CV Mosby

Atchison DA (1987) Effect of defocus on visual field measurement. *Ophthalmic and Physiological Optics*, 7: 259

Autzen T, Work K (1990) The effect of learning and age on short-term fluctuation and mean sensitivity of automated static perimetry. *Acta Ophthalmologica*, 68: 327

Balazsi AG, Rootman J, Drance SM, Schulzer M, Douglas GR (1984) The effect of age on the nerve fibre population of the human optic nerve. *American Journal of Ophthalmology*, 97: 760

Cahill KV, Burns JA, Weber PA (1987) The effects of blepharoptosis on the field of vision. *Ophthalmic and Plastic Reconstructive Surgery*, **3**: 121

Donahue S (1998) Lens holder artifact simulating glaucomatous defect in automated perimetry. *Archives of Ophthalmology*, **116**: 1681

Edgar D, Crabb D, Rudnicka A, Lawrenson J, Guttridge N, O'Brien C (1999) Effects of dipivefrin and pilocarpine on pupil diameter, automated perimetry and LogMAR acuity. *Graefe's Archives of Clinical Experimental Ophthalmology*, **237**: 117

Federici T, Meyer D, Lininger L (1999) Correlation of the vision-related functional impairment associated with blepharoptosis and the impact of blepharoptosis surgery. *Ophthalmology*, **106**: 1705

Gonzalez de la Rosa M, Pareja A (1997) Influence of the fatigue effect on the mean deviation measurement in perimetry. *European Journal of Ophthalmology*, **7**: 29

Guthauser U, Flammer J, Niesel P (1987) Relationship between cataract density and visual field damage. *Documenta Ophthalmologica Proceedings Series*, **49**: 39

Guthauser V, Flammer J (1988) Quantifying visual field damage caused by cataract. *American Journal of Ophthalmology*, **106**: 480

Haas A, Flammer J, Schneider U (1986) Influence of age on the visual fields of normal subjects. *American Journal of Ophthalmology*, **101**: 199

Henson D, Earlam R (1995) Correcting lens system for perimetry. *Ophthalmic and Physiological Optics*, **15**: 59

Henson DB, Morris EJ (1993) Effect of uncorrected refractive errors upon central visual field testing. *Ophthalmic and Physiological Optics*, **13**: 339

Hudson C, Wild JM, O'Neill EC (1994) Fatigue effects during a single session of automated static threshold perimetry. *Investigative Ophthalmology and Visual Science*, **35**: 268

Johnson CA, Adamo AJ, Lewis RA (1989) Evidence for a neural basis of age-related visual field loss in normal observers. *Investigative Ophthalmology*, **30**: 2056

Katz J, Sommer A, Witt K (1991) Reliability of visual field results over repeated testing. *Ophthalmology*, **98**: 70

Keane JR (1977) Hysterical hemianopia: the missing half field defect. *Archives of Ophthalmology*, **97**: 865

Klingele J, Kaiser HJ, Hatt M (1995) Automated perimetry in ptosis and blepharochalasis. *Klinische Monatsblaetter fuer Augenheilkunde*, **206**: 401

Lindermuth KA, Skuta GL, Rabbani R, Musch DC (1989) Effect of pupillary constriction on automated perimetry in normal eyes. *Ophthalmology*, **96**: 1289

Meyer D, Stern J, Lininger L (1993) Evaluating the visual field effects of blepharoptosis using automated static perimetry. *Ophthalmology*, **100**: 651

Mikelberg FS, Drance SM, Schutzer M, Wijsman K (1987) The effect of miosis on visual field indices. *Documenta Ophthalmologica Proceedings Series*, **49**: 645

Nordmann JP, Denis P, Nguer Y, Mouton-Chopin D, Saraux H (1994) Static threshold visual field in glaucoma with the Fastpac algorithm of the Humphrey Field Analyzer. Is the gain in examination time offset by any loss of information? *European Journal of Ophthalmology*, **4**: 105

O'Brien C, Poinoosawmy D, Wu J, Hitchings R (1994) Evaluation of the Humphrey FASTPAC threshold program in glaucoma. *British Journal of Ophthalmology*, **78**: 516

Rowe FJ (1998) Visual field analysis with Humphrey automated perimetry. Parts I and II. *Eye News*, **4**(6); **5**(1).

Smith T, Baker R (1987) Perimetric findings in functional disorders using automated techniques. *Ophthalmology*, **94**: 1562

Spaeth GL (1980) The management of cataract in patients with glaucoma: a comparative study I. *Transactions of the Ophthalmological Societies of the UK*, **100**: 195

Steel SE, Mackie SW, Walsh G (1996) Visual field defects due to spectacle frames: their prediction and relationship to UK driving standards. *Ophthalmic and Physiological Optics*, **16**: 95

Webster A, Luff A, Canning C, Elkington A (1993) The effect of pilocarpine on the glaucomatous visual field. *British Journal of Ophthalmology*, **77**: 721

Weinreb RN, Perlman JP (1986) The effect of refractive correction on automated perimetric thresholds. *American Journal of Ophthalmology*, **101**: 706

Werner EB, Adelson A, Krupin T (1988) Effect of patient experience on the results of automated perimetry in clinically stable glaucoma patients. *Ophthalmology*, **95**: 764

Wild JM, Searle AE, Dengler-Harles M, O'Neill EC (1991) Long-term follow-up of baseline learning and fatigue effects in the automated perimetry of glaucoma and ocular hypertensive patients. *Acta Ophthalmologica*, **69**: 210

Zalta AH (1989) Lens rim artefact in automated threshold perimetry. *Ophthalmology*, **96**: 1302

Further reading

Thompson HS (1985) Functional visual loss. *American Journal of Ophthalmology*, **100**: 209

Chapter 14

Glossary of terms in visual field assessment

24-2 programme
The 24-2 full threshold programme tests the central 24 degrees of the visual field but including the nasal field to 30 degrees, and tests 54 points with a 6 degree spaced grid offset from the vertical and horizontal meridians.

30-2 programme
The 30-2 full threshold programme tests the central 30 degrees of the visual field and tests 76 points with a 6 degree spaced grid offset from the vertical and horizontal meridians.

Acalculia
A form of aphasia characterised by the inability to perform simple mathematical problems.

Achromatopsia
Complete loss of colour perception.

Agnosia
The patient cannot identify previously familiar objects by sight despite adequate visual acuity, nor learn to identify new objects by sight alone. When the patient is allowed to feel, smell or listen, the object can be identified.

Agraphia
Impaired writing ability.

Alexia
Loss of reading ability in previously literate persons. Global alexia includes an inability to read numbers, letters, symbols and words.

Altitudinal visual field defect
This involves two quadrants of either the superior or inferior visual field and precisely respects the horizontal meridian.

Anton's syndrome
A small minority of patients with cortical blindness behave as though they are not aware of their deficit and insist that they can see.

Aphasia
Aphasia is a loss of ability to produce correct speech.

Apostilb
An absolute unit of light measurement equal to 0.1 millilamberts.

Arcuate visual field defect
This is caused by selective damage to the superior or inferior retinal nerve fibre bundles with a narrow defect temporally but spreading out on the nasal side and extending to the horizontal meridian.

Artefact
An artificial defect.

Background illumination
The background illumination is set at 31.5 apostilb.

Binocular
Both eyes.

Box plot
The entire box plot from tail to tail represents the entire visual field responses. The height of the various portions of the box plot indicates the degree to which different points are more severely affected than others, or the variability in the amount of involvement of the various points. The lower and upper tails each represent 15% of points and the centre box, 70%. The lower tail represents the worst points (lowest decibel values) and the upper tail represents the best points (highest decibel values).

Caecocentral scotoma
A caecocentral scotoma extends from fixation to the blind spot.

Calibration
Initial set-up of perimeter settings, such as background and stimuli intensities.

Campimetry
Visual field assessment using a flat surface, e.g. Bjerrum screen or Friedmann.

Candela
A unit of luminance intensity.

Cecocentral scotoma
See caecocentral scotoma

Central scotoma
A central scotoma involves only fixation.

Central visual field
The visual field within the central 30 degrees of fixation.

Centrocaecal scotoma
See caecocentral scotoma

Change analysis printout
This will give a statistical evaluation of change in visual field over time. Global indices are summarised in chronological order and a box plot is used to illustrate the visual field responses graphically .

Checkerboard visual field defect
Crossed quadrant hemianopia.

Cog wheel movements
Episodic rotations with pursuit movements.

Cogan's sign
A conjugate movement of the eyes to the side opposite the lesion on forced lid closure.

Colour perimetry
Visual field assessment with coloured targets presented on a white background or on a coloured background.

Congruous
Post chiasm visual field defects that are similar in extent in either eye.

Contralateral
Referring to the opposite side.

Corrected pattern standard deviation
This combines the pattern standard deviation and the short term fluctuation to take into consideration any intratest variability.

Cortical blindness
Cortical blindness is associated with bilateral complete or severe hemianopia with no detectable peripheral visual field. Visual acuity is light perception only or worse.

Cortical magnification
Over half of visual cortex is devoted to the central 10 degrees of nerve fibres and this is termed cortical magnification.

Decibel
Decibel values equal $\frac{1}{10}$ th of a log unit (10 decibels equals 1 log unit) and allow larger numbers to be expressed as smaller numerical units (0 decibels = 1000 apostilb = 300 cd/m^2).

Defect grid
Shows the difference of the patient responses to those expected from a normal field.

Dysphasia
Dysphasia is a language disorder whereby there is an inability to speak words which one has in mind or to think of correct words, or an inability to understand spoken or written words.

Esterman programme
The Esterman programme is used for DVLA driving visual field assessments and may be performed as a binocular or monocular test.

False negative
Throughout the test, a stimulus is projected at a level above threshold at a point which has already had a positive response to a certain decibel value. The patient should therefore respond to this; however, if there is no response, this is recorded as a false negative.

False positive
During the test, the projection device is at times moved, or clicks without presenting a stimulus. Should the patient respond despite the absence of a stimulus, this is recorded as a false positive.

Fastpac test
The stimulus intensity is increased in 3 decibel steps until recorded and then decreased to below the threshold level and increased again, in 3 decibel steps, until recorded, to confirm the threshold level at that point.

Fixation loss
Stimuli are periodically presented in the patient's blind spot area to which there should be no response. Should the patient's fixation alter, a response will be made to the stimuli and this is recorded as a fixation loss.

Fluctuation
See short term and long term fluctuation

Full from prior threshold test
The last test to be performed is recalled and the threshold levels for each point from the last test used as starting levels for the current test. The stimuli are initially started at a level 2 decibels higher than the previous threshold, and the test then continues as for a full threshold programme.

Full threshold test
The stimulus intensity is increased in 4 decibel steps until recorded and then decreased to below the threshold level and increased again, in 2 decibel steps, until recorded, to confirm the threshold level at that point.

Functional
Patient shows signs or symptoms of a visual disorder, but careful examination fails to reveal any evidence of structural or physiological abnormalities.

Gaze tracking
A measure of gaze direction each time a stimulus is presented.

Glaucoma change probability printout
The first and second field results are combined as an average and consecutive fields are then compared to this for progression of the condition. The printout provides a greyscale of the current test, the total deviation plot, the change from the average baseline plot and its associated probability plot.

Glaucoma hemifield test
This compares areas of the superior field with corresponding areas of the inferior field to determine whether the response to stimuli is comparable in the superior and inferior areas of the visual field.

Global indices
These include mean deviation, pattern standard deviation, corrected pattern standard deviation and short term fluctuation.

Graphaesthesia
A tactual inability to recognise writing.

Greyscale
Provides an immediate view of the visual field and a scale shows the corresponding values of the greyscale in apostilbs and decibels. Each change in the greyscale tone is equivalent to a 5 decibel change in threshold.

Hemiachromatopsia
Colour loss in the contralateral visual hemifield.

Hemianopia
A hemianopia is a complete defect involving one half of the visual field.

Hemiparesis
Hemiparesis is a paralysis affecting only one side of the body.

Heteronymous
A heteronymous visual field defect involves opposite sides of the visual field.

Hill of vision
A map of the visual field in three dimensions

Homonymous
A homonymous visual field defect involves the same side of the visual field in each eye.

Incongruous
Post chiasm visual field defects that are dissimilar in extent in either eye.

Infrathreshold
The stimulus intensity is below the level at which it can be seen by the patient.

Ipsilateral
Referring to the same side.

Isopter
The boundary between regions of invisibility and visibility is the isopter, a perimeter line that connects all points at which the stimulus has been seen.

Kinetic perimetry
In kinetic threshold perimetry, a stimulus is moved from an area in which it is not seen (infrathreshold) into a region where it is visible (suprathreshold).

Learning curve
The learning curve involves learning to respond consistently during the test; thus the visual field assessment improves with experience.

Lens rim defect
Poorly positioned lenses will interfere with visual perception as stimuli will not be seen by the patient if blocked by a poorly positioned lens.

Light intensity
Light intensity is expressed in apostilbs, an absolute unit of light measurement: 1 apostilb is equal to 0.1 millilambert.

Long-term fluctuation
Variability of visual field sensitivity between visual field examinations.

Luminance units
Luminance units are candelas per square metre (cd/m^2).

Luminance values
Values are plotted at different points within the field of vision to give sensitivities at those points across the visual field.

Macular sparing
Hemianopia without involvement of the macular visual field.

Macular splitting
Hemianopia with involvement of the macular visual field.

Map of isopters
This is used to document the area of visual field and isopters are assessed with targets of differing size and luminance.

Mean deviation
The mean deviation is the overall departure of the average deviation of the visual field result from that expected of a normal field of the same age group.

Meyer's loop
Passing from the lateral geniculate body, the nerve fibres of the inferior bundle are at first directed anteriorly and laterally superior to and around the inferior horn of the lateral ventricle to form Meyer's loop.

Miosis
Constriction of the pupil.

Monocular
One eye.

Nasal step
Visual field defect occurring in the nasal visual field with clear demarcation along the horizontal meridian.

Numeric grid
Provides the patient responses at each point in decibel values.

Ocular media
The ocular media comprise all 'clear' structures of the eye through which light rays pass to reach the retina.

Overview printouts
These printouts present each field in succession with the greyscale, total deviation and probability plots for the total and pattern deviations. The global indices are also included.

Papillomacular bundle
A high percentage of nerve fibres arise from the macular area of the retina and pass directly to the optic disc.

Paracentral scotoma
A paracentral scotoma involves an area of visual field away from fixation.

Pattern deviation plot
The pattern deviation is similar to the total deviation but adjusts the field according to any overall depression or elevation of response values in order to highlight any localised areas of visual loss that may have been masked.

Pattern standard deviation
The pattern standard deviation is determined by the variation from the normal hill of vision.

Perimeter
Equipment to measure the visual field.

Perimetry
Visual field assessment using a curved background, e.g. Goldmann or Humphrey perimeter.

Peripheral visual field
The visual field extending from the central 30 degrees out to 50 degrees superiorly, 60 degrees nasally, 70 degrees inferiorly and 100 degrees temporally.

Pie in the sky
Term used to describe a partial superior homonymous quadrantanopia occurring with temporal lobe lesions involving Meyer's loop of optic radiation nerve fibres.

Prosopagnosia
Patients no longer recognise the faces of previously familiar persons, nor learn newly encountered faces.

Quadrantanopia
This is a complete defect involving a quadrant of each visual field.

Reliability indices
Test reliability is monitored by determination of fixation losses, false positive and false negative responses.

Riddoch phenomenon
See stato-kinetic dissociation

Scotoma
A scotoma is an absolute or relative area of depressed visual function surrounded by normal vision.

Screening
Screening programmes involve the use of suprathreshold tests where the visual field is assessed using targets of brightness level above that which would be expected to be seen for the age of the patient.

Sector visual field defect
These visual field defects start as small scotomas on the temporal side of the visual field and end as complete sectorial loss.

Sensitivity
The sensitivity of the visual field is expressed in luminance or light intensity units.

Short-term fluctuation
This is to monitor reliability of responses during a test. Ten pre-selected points are checked twice to determine reliability of response.

SITA
Swedish Interactive Thresholding Algorithm.

Simultanagnosia
Patients are unable to recognise multiple elements in a visual presentation, in that one object or some elements of a scene can be appreciated, but not the scene as a whole.

Single field analysis printout
Provides six field plots, a greyscale, a numeric grid plus a total deviation grid and pattern standard deviation grid with their relevant probability plots.

Static perimetry
A target of known brightness at suprathreshold level is flashed on briefly within the boundaries of the patient's visual field.

Stato-kinetic dissociation
Defects present on automated perimetry tend to be more extensive than those present on manual perimetry (also known as Riddoch phenomenon).

Statpac
Statpac is the statistical program used to analyse the data from single, or multiple, visual field assessments using threshold programmes.

Suprathreshold
The stimulus is at a level at which it can be seen by the patient.

Temporal crescent visual field defect
Monocular defect in the extreme temporal visual field.

Three in one printout
Provides a greyscale, a defect depth grid and a numeric grid.

Threshold
The sensitivity of each specific area of the visual field tested.

Total deviation
The total deviation is the deviation of patient responses from normal values.

Visual field
The visual field is produced by retinal stimulation of each eye and relates to what is seen by the individual, i.e. the perceived vision of an individual. The normal monocular visual field extends 50 degrees superiorly, 60 degrees nasally, 70 degrees inferiorly and 100 degrees temporally.

Visual neglect
Neglect is a multifaceted disorder manifesting itself within different sensory domains and reference frames, and cannot be explained by a simple retinotopic visual deficit. Even when a patient directs their eyes to one side (usually the left), targets to the left of the body midline are ignored.

Visual pathway
The afferent visual pathway consists of the retinal ganglion cells, optic disc, optic nerve, optic chiasm, optic tract, lateral geniculate body, optic radiations and striate visual cortex.

Wedge defect
These visual field defects start as small scotomas on the temporal side of the visual field and end as complete sectorial loss.

Index